BRUCE H. THIERS, MD, Consulting Editor

theclinics.com

DERMATOLOGIC CLINICS

Photodynamic Therapy

MICHAEL H. GOLD, MD
Guest Editor

January 2007 • Volume 25 • Number 1

SAUNDERS

An Imprint of Elsevier, Inc.
PHILADELPHIA   LONDON   TORONTO   MONTREAL   SYDNEY   TOKYO

W.B. SAUNDERS COMPANY
A Division of Elsevier Inc.

Elsevier Inc. • 1600 John F. Kennedy Blvd., Suite 1800 • Philadelphia, Pennsylvania 19103-2899

http://www.theclinics.com

DERMATOLOGIC CLINICS
January 2007
Editor: Alexandra Gavenda

Volume 25, Number 1
ISSN 0733-8635
ISBN 1-4160-4304-7
978-1-4160-4304-1

The ideas and opinions expressed in *Dermatologic Clinics* do not necessarily reflect those of the Publisher. The Publisher does not assume any responsibility for any injury and/or damage to persons or property arising out of or related to any use of the material contained in this periodical. The reader is advised to check the appropriate medical literature and the product information currently provided by the manu-facturer of each drug to be administered to verify the dosage, the method and duration of administration, or contraindications. It is the responsibility of the treating physician or other health care professional, re-lying on independent experience and knowledge of the patient, to determine drug dosages and the best treatment for the patient. Mention of any product in this issue should not be construed as endorsement by the contributors, editors, or the Publisher of the product or manufacturers' claims.

Dermatologic Clinics (ISSN 0733-8635) is published quarterly by Elsevier Inc., 360 Park Avenue South, New York, NY 10010-1710. Months of publication are January, April, July, and October. Business and edi-torial offices: 1600 John F. Kennedy Blvd., Suite 1800, Philadelphia, PA 19103-2899. Customer service of-fice: 6277 Sea Harbor Drive, Orlando, FL 32887-4800. Periodicals postage paid at New York, NY, and additional mailing offices. Subscription prices are USD 231 per year for US individuals, USD 356 per year for US institutions, USD 270 per year for Canadian individuals, USD 416 per year for Canadian institu-tions, USD 297 per year for international individuals, USD 416 per year for international institutions, USD 110 per year for US students, USD 149 per year for Canadian students, and USD 149 per year for international students. International air speed delivery is included in all *Clinics* subscription prices. All prices are subject to change without notice. POSTMASTER: Send address changes to *Dermatologic Clinics*, Elsevier Periodicals Customer Service, 6277 Sea Harbor Drive, Orlando, FL 32887-4800. **Customer Ser-vice: 1-800-654-2452 (US). From outside of the US, call 1-407-345-4000. E-mail: hhspcs@harcourt.com**.

Reprints. For copies of 100 or more, of articles in this publication, please contact the Commercial Re-prints Department, Elsevier Inc., 360 Park Avenue South, New York, New York 10010-1710. Tel.: (212) 633-3813; Fax: (212) 462-1935; Email: repritns@elsevier.com.

The *Dermatologic Clinics* is covered in *Index Medicus*, *Current Contents/Clinical Medicine*, *Excerpta Medica*, *Chemical Abstracts*, and *ISI/BIOMED*.

Printed in the United States of America.

CONSULTING EDITOR

BRUCE H. THIERS, MD, Professor and Chair, Department of Dermatology, Medical University of South Carolina, Charleston, South Carolina

GUEST EDITOR

MICHAEL H. GOLD, MD, Medical Director, Gold Skin Care Center, Tennessee Clinical Research Center; and Clinical Assistant Professor, Vanderbilt University Medical School, Vanderbilt University Nursing School, Nashville, Tennessee

CONTRIBUTORS

MACRENE ALEXIADES-ARMENAKAS, MD, PhD, Assistant Clinical Professor, Yale University School of Medicine, New Haven, Connecticut

ROBERT BISSONNETTE, MD, FRCPC, Innovaderm Research, Montréal, Quebec, Canada

JONATHAN E. BLUME, MD, Clinical Assistant Instructor, Department of Dermatology, State University of New York at Buffalo, Buffalo, New York

DORE J. GILBERT, MD, Medical Director, Newport Dermatology and Laser Associates, Newport Beach; and Associate Clinical Professor of Dermatology, University of California, Irvine, Irvine, California

MICHAEL H. GOLD, MD, Medical Director, Gold Skin Care Center, Tennessee Clinical Research Center; and Clinical Assistant Professor, Vanderbilt University Medical School, Vanderbilt University Nursing School, Nashville, Tennessee

MITCHEL P. GOLDMAN, MD, Medical Director, La Jolla Spa MD, La Jolla; and Associate Clinical Professor of Dermatology and Medicine, University of California, San Diego, California

MICHAL S. KALISIAK, MD, Division of Dermatology and Cutaneous Sciences, University of Alberta, Edmonton, Alberta, Canada

ALI MOIIN, MD, Clinical Associate Professor, Department of Dermatology, Wayne State University School of Medicine, Detroit, Michigan

COLIN A. MORTON, MBChB, MD, FRCP, Consultant in Dermatology, Forth Valley Dermatology Centre, Stirling Royal Infirmary, Stirling, United Kingdom

MARK S. NESTOR, MD, PhD, Center for Cosmetic Enhancement, Aventura, Florida

PAVAN K. NOOTHETI, MD, Cosmetic Dermatologist, La Jolla Spa MD, La Jolla, California

ALLAN R. OSEROFF, MD, PhD, Professor and Lawrence P. and Joan Castellani Family Endowed Chair in Dermatology, Department of Dermatology, Roswell Park Cancer Institute; and Department of Dermatology, State University of New York at Buffalo, Buffalo, New York

JAGGI RAO, MD, FRCPC, Division of Dermatology and Cutaneous Sciences, University of Alberta, Edmonton, Alberta, Canada

DONALD F. RICHEY, MD, North Valley Dermatology Center, Chico, California

ROLF-MARKUS SZEIMIES, MD, PhD, Associate Professor, Department of Dermatology, Regensburg University Hospital, Regensburg, Germany

AMY FORMAN TAUB, MD, Clinical Instructor, Department of Dermatology, Northwestern University Medical School, Chicago; and Founder and Director, Advanced Dermatology, Lincolnshire, Illinois

CONTENTS

long-term consequences. The use of photodynamic therapy (PDT) recently has been described as a treatment option for intractable HS. The clinical trials that are associated with PDT and HS are reviewed, and thoughts about the probable mechanisms of actions of this therapy are given. PDT should be considered in patients who have severe HS.

Photodynamic Therapy: Other Uses
Amy Forman Taub

Mainstream uses for photodynamic therapy (PDT) in dermatology include nonmelanoma skin cancer and its precursors, acne vulgaris, photorejuvenation, and hidradenitis suppurativa. Many other dermatologic entities have been treated with PDT, including psoriasis, lichen planus, lichen sclerosus, scleroderma, cutaneous T cell lymphoma, alopecia areata, verruca vulgaris, Darier's disease and tinea infections. Nondermatologic applications include anal and vulvar carcinoma, palliation of metastatic breast cancer to skin, Barrett's esophagus, and macular degeneration of the retina. PDT also has found to be useful in immunologic and inflammatory disorders, neoplasias other than skin cancer, and infections. The ability of this treatment to hone in on dysplastic epithelial and endothelial cells while retaining viability of surrounding tissue is its key feature because this leads to specific tumor destruction with cosmesis and function of the target organ intact.

Incorporating Photodynamic Therapy into a Medical and Cosmetic Dermatology Practice
Dore J. Gilbert

Effective in the treatment of a growing variety of skin conditions, photodynamic therapy (PDT) with 5-aminolevulinic acid (ALA) is rising rapidly in popularity among both practitioners and patients, despite the fact that many applications are not yet cleared by the Food and Drug Administration. Because of its versatility, safety, efficacy, cosmetic benefits, and potential financial advantages, ALA-PDT may soon be a mainstay in many clinical settings. This article provides an overview of this easy-to-use treatment modality and a guide to implementing ALA-PDT into practice, including pretreatment and posttreatment protocols and guidelines for managing side effects.

Photodynamic Therapy in Dermatology: the Next Five Years
Michael H. Gold

Photodynamic therapy (PDT) has had a rapid insurgence into the dermatologic armamentarium of clinicians from all over the world. Its use in actinic keratoses and in nonmelanoma skin cancers is well described. Additional uses, including its use in the treatment of photorejuvenation and acne vulgaris and related disorders, are gaining more widespread use. More recent descriptions, including its potential use as a chemoprevention agent, warrant further investigations and discussions. PDT is a global treatment modality and physicians and investigators must view the therapy as such, and use the best photosensitizer for the best indication, and continue to evaluate new approaches to maximize the use of PDT in dermatology.

FORTHCOMING ISSUES

April 2007

Drug Actions, Reactions, and Interactions
James Q. Del Rosso, DO, *Guest Editor*

July 2007

Pigmentary Disorders
Torello Lotti, MD, *Guest Editor*

October 2007

**Cutaneous Receptors: Clinical Implications
and Therapeutic Relevance**
Ronni Wolf, MD, and Batya Davidovici, MD,
Guest Editors

RECENT ISSUES

October 2006

**The Skin and HIV/AIDS:
A Quarter Century Update**
Roy Colven, MD, *Guest Editor*

July 2006

Nail Disorders and their Management
Aditya K. Gupta, MD, PhD, FRCP(C), and
Robert Baran, MD, *Guest Editors*

April 2006

Women's Dermatology
Kathryn Schwarzenberger, MD, *Guest Editor*

THE CLINICS ARE NOW AVAILABLE ONLINE!

Access your subscription at
http://www.theclinics.com

SINGLETON HOSPITAL
STAFF LIBRARY

DERMATOLOGIC
CLINICS

ELSEVIER
SAUNDERS

Dermatol Clin 25 (2007) xi

Preface

Michael H. Gold, MD
Guest Editor

Photodynamic therapy (PDT) has become one of the fastest growing therapeutic modalities over the past several years. Clinicians from all over the world are finding new and exciting uses for PDT in their clinical practices.

I am honored to be the guest editor of this issue of *Dermatologic Clinics*, focusing on the global field of PDT. An outstanding group of authors with extensive knowledge in the use of the two available photosensitizers, 5-aminolevulinic acid and the methyl ester derivative, have prepared the context for the following pages, which provides the reader with the history of PDT, where PDT had its early successes, where PDT is now, and where PDT will be in the near future.

PDT has its origins in the treatment of actinic keratoses (AKs) and nonmelanoma skin cancer, and will continue to be a major contributor in the therapy of these disorders. Our experts have reviewed the medical literature and present to the reader the evidence-based medicine that has shown the effectiveness of PDT in treating these disorders. Recently, new information has arisen showing that PDT can be used to treat the signs of photorejuvenation, and these data are also presented. PDT is also routinely used to treat moderate to severe inflammatory acne vulgaris and other disorders of sebaceous glands—newer uses, but very important nonetheless. Other novel uses of PDT are also presented, showing the versatility of this therapy for everyday use in clinical practice.

I hope readers enjoy this text. It has been a pleasure working with these outstanding contributors.

Michael H. Gold, MD
Gold Skin Care Center
Tennessee Clinical Research Center
2000 Richard Jones Road
Suite 220
Nashville, TN 37215, USA

Vanderbilt University School of Medicine
Vanderbilt University Nursing School
Nashville, TN 37215, USA

E-mail address: goldskin@goldskincare.com

doi:10.1016/j.det.2006.09.016

ELSEVIER
SAUNDERS

Dermatol Clin 25 (2007) 1–4

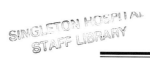

DERMATOLOGIC
CLINICS

Introduction to Photodynamic Therapy: Early Experience

Michael H. Gold, MD[a,b,*]

[a]*Gold Skin Care Center, Tennessee Clinical Research Center, 200 Richard Jones Road, Suite 200, Nashville, TN 37215, USA*
[b]*Vanderbilt University Medical School, Vanderbilt University Nursing School, Nashville, TN 37215, USA*

The use of photodynamic therapy (PDT) with appropriate photosensitizers has grown steadily over the past several years, prompting this issue of *the Dermatologic Clinics*. I am grateful to the publishers for allowing me the opportunity to edit this issue on a field of study that truly is close to my heart. I have been involved in the United States' study of PDT since its introduction in the late 1990s. I have had the opportunity to study PDT on a variety of dermatologic disorders, including actinic keratoses (AK), photorejuvenation, inflammatory acne vulgaris, sebaceous gland hyperplasia, and hidradenitis suppurativa. I also have been fortunate to collaborate with other investigators from all over the world to learn how they use PDT, how they view the field, and how PDT is working in countries all over the world.

The history of PDT can be traced to the early 1900s. Raab [1] first reported, in 1900, that paramecia cells (*Paramecium caudatum*) were unaffected when exposed to acridine orange or light, but that they died within 2 hours when exposed to both at the same time. Von Tappeiner and Jodblauer [2], in 1904, first described the term "photodynamic effect" when they showed an oxygen-consuming reaction process in protozoa after aniline dyes were applied with fluorescence. In 1905, Jesionek and Von Tappeiner [3] described experiences with topical 5% eosin. Topical 5% eosin was used as a photosensitizer with artificial light to treat nonmelanoma skin cancers, lupus vulgaris, and condylomata lata in humans successfully. It was postulated that the eosin, in a manner similar to the acridine orange studies, once incorporated into cells, could produce a cytotoxic reaction when exposed to a light source and oxygen. These were the first reports of PDT in patients and led the way to what PDT has become today.

After these initial descriptions of eosin and acridine orange use as photosensitizers, researchers turned their attention to the study of porphyrins. In 1911, Hausman [4] reported on the use of hematoporphyrin. He successfully showed that light-activated hematoporphyrin could photosensitize guinea pigs and mice. In 1913, Meyer-Betz [5] injected himself with hematoporphyrin, and noticed that, when the areas he injected were exposed to light, they became swollen and painful. Unfortunately, the phototoxic reaction lasted for 2 months, which created difficulty for its regular use as a photosensitizer. In 1942, Auler and Banzer [6] showed that hematoporphyrin concentrated more in certain dermatologic tumors than in their surrounding tissues; when fluoresced, the tumors were necrotic, which demonstrated the photodynamic response of hematoporphyrin. Figge and his associates [7] later

Dr. Gold is a consultant for Dusa Pharmaceuticals, speaks on their behalf, receives honoraria, and performs research on their behalf. Dr. Gold also is a consultant for numerous pharmaceutical and device companies and performs research on their behalf.

* Gold Skin Care Center, Tennessee Clinical Research Center, 2000 Richard Jones Road, Suite 220, Nashville, TN 37215.

E-mail address: goldskin@goldskincare.com

reported that hematoporphyrin also was absorbed selectively into other cells, including embryonic, traumatized skin, and neoplastic areas.

The principles of PDT in human cancer cells had been established. A proper photosensitizer, in this case hematoporphyrin, could be concentrated in the cancerous cells, and when activated by a proper light source in the presence of oxygen, would be cytotoxic to these cells. In 1978, Dougherty and colleagues [8] presented research with a new photosensitizer, hematoporphyrin purified derivative (HPD). HPD was a complex mixture of porphyrin subunits and by-products. They showed that HPD could be used successfully to treat cutaneous malignancies, with red light being the primary light source. Systemic HPD became the standard for PDT research, and a variety of medical uses—oncologic and nononcologic—emerged for PDT (Box 1).

Because of the unique nature of the skin and its accessibility to be studied with natural light or artificial light sources, dermatologic research became a prime focus for PDT study. HPD, however, remained phototoxic in the skin for several months, which makes its practical use in dermatology difficult. In 1990, Kennedy and his group [9] introduced the first topical porphyrin derivative, known as aminolevulinic acid (ALA). This photosensitizing prodrug had the ability to penetrate the stratum corneum of the skin and be absorbed by actinically damaged skin cells, as well as nonmelanoma skin cancer cells and pilosebaceous units. Their group described the PDT reaction of ALA; once incorporated into a particular cell, ALA is converted to its active form, protoporphyrin IX (PpIX). ALA, the natural precursor of PpIX in the heme pathway. ALA is the prodrug photosensitizing agent; PpIX is the photosensitizer. PpIX has been shown to be photoactivated by a variety of lasers and light sources (Fig. 1). The absorption spectrum of PpIX, with peak absorption bands identified in the blue light and red light spectrums, is shown in Fig. 1. Smaller peaks of energy, in between these major absorption bands, also are identified; this has become important and will become apparent as ALA-PDT moves into the twenty-first century [10].

The heme biosynthetic pathway (Fig. 2) is maintained under a close feedback loop apparatus, which does not allow for buildup of heme or its precursors, such as PpIX, in tissues. Exogenous ALA-forming PpIX is cleared from the body much more rapidly than is its predecessor

---

Box 1. Uses of photodynamic therapy

Medical uses for PDT
Malignancies
   Lung
   Esophagus
   Colon
   Peritoneum
   Pleura
   Gastrointestinal tract
   Brain
   Eye
   Skin

Nononcologic conditions
   Atherosclerosis
   Infectious diseases
   Rheumatoid arthritis

Dermatologic entities that are treated with ALA-PDT
   Cutaneous T-cell lymphoma
   Kaposi's sarcoma
   Malignant melanoma
   Keratoacanthoma
   Extramammary Paget's disease
   Acne vulgaris
   Sebaceous gland hyperplasia
   Hidradenitis suppurativa
   Psoriasis vulgaris
   Verrucae vulgaris
   Molluscum contagiosum
   Actinic chelitis
   Hirsutism
   Alopecia areata
   Photorejuvenation/photoaging

Adapted from Gold MH, editor. Photodynamic therapy. In: Cutaneous and cosmetic laser surgery. 1st edition. Elsevier; 2006. p. 277–92; with permission.

---

photosensitizer, HPD. Therefore, the potential for phototoxicity from ALA-induced PpIX, is much reduced—to days instead of several months. Also, ALA penetrates only actinically damaged skin, which increases the specificity of ALA-PDT.

ALA-PDT has taken on two separate identities since Kennedy and colleagues' introduction of topically applied ALA. In the United States, research has centered on 20% 5-ALA (Levulan Kerastick, Dusa Pharmaceuticals, Wilmington, Massachusetts) and

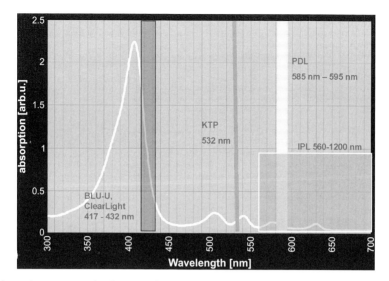

Fig. 1. PpIX absorption spectrum in vivo. IPL, intense pulse light; KTP, potassium titanyl phosphate; PDL, pulse dye laser. (*From* Nestor MS, Gold MH, Kauvar AN, et al. The use of photodynamic therapy in dermatology: results of a consensus conference. J Drugs Dermatol 2006;5:140–54; with permission.)

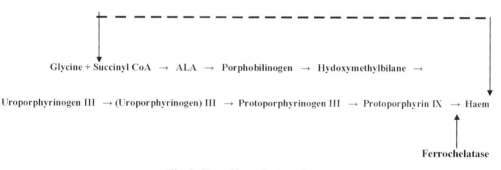

Fig. 2. Heme biosynthetic pathway.

its ability to treat AK, photorejuvenation, inflammatory acne vulgaris, sebaceous gland hyperplasia, and hidradenitis predominantly. In Europe, research has centered on the methyl ester of 5-ALA (Metvix, PhotoCure ASA, Oslo, Norway) and its uses in treating nonmelanoma skin cancers and AK. Interest in photorejuvenation and inflammatory acne vulgaris is at its infancy [10]. This issue explores the various drugs, the various indications for each drug, and allows the reader the opportunity to determine if PDT can play a vital role in his/her daily practice of medicine.

This issue highlights some of the brightest minds that are involved in the study of PDT from all over the world. PDT is a global subspecialty, and it is important to view it in this manner. PDT has several uses; the primary ones are highlighted by investigators who share the passion that I have for PDT. As I describe at the end of this issue, all of the indications and uses for PDT are new and exciting; however, the potential role that PDT has as a chemoprevention therapy is huge, and something that I cannot stress to colleagues enough. I hope that you enjoy this issue and I hope that it excites you to enter the world of PDT.

References

[1] Raab O. Ueber die wirkung fluoreszierenden stoffe auf infusorien. Z Biol 1900;39:524–6.
[2] Von Tappeiner H, Jodblauer A. Uber die wirkung der photodynamischen (fluorescierenden) staffe auf protozoan und enzyme. Dtsch Arch Klin Med 1904;80:427–87.

[3] Jesionek A, Von Tappeiner H. Behandlung der haut-carcinome nut fluorescierenden stoffen. Dtsch Arch Klin Med 1905;85:223–7.

[4] Hausman W. Die sensibilisierende wirkung des hamatoporphyrins. Biochem Zeit 1911;276–316.

[5] Meyer-Betz F. Untersuchungen uber die bioloische (photodynamische) wirkung des hamatoporphyrins und anderer derivative des blut-und gallenfarbstoffs. Dtsch Arch Klin Med 1913;112:476–503.

[6] Auler H, Banzer G. Untersuchungen ueber die rolle der porphyrine bei geschwulstkranken menschen und tieren. Z Krebsforsch 1942;53:65–8.

[7] Figge FHJ, Weiland GS, Manganiello LDJ. Cancer detection and therapy. Affinity of neoplastic embryonic and traumatized tissue for porphyrins and metalloporphyrins. Proc Soc Exp Biol Med 1948;68:640.

[8] Dougherty TJ, Kaufman JE, Goldfarb A, et al. Photoradiation therapy for the treatment of malignant tumors. Cancer Res 1978;38:2628–35.

[9] Kennedy JC, Pottier RH, Pross DC, et al. Photodynamic therapy with endogenous protoporphyrin IX: basic principles and present clinical experiences. J Photochem Photobiol B 1990;6:143–8.

[10] Gold MH, Goldman MP. 5-Aminolevulinic acid photodynamic therapy: where we have been and where we are going. Dermatol Surg 2004;30:1077–84.

DERMATOLOGIC
CLINICS

Dermatol Clin 25 (2007) 5–14

Aminolevulinic Acid Photodynamic Therapy for Skin Cancers

Jonathan E. Blume, MD[a], Allan R. Oseroff, MD, PhD[a,b],*

[a]Department of Dermatology, State University of New York at Buffalo, Elm and Carlton Streets, Buffalo, NY 14263, USA
[b]Department of Dermatology, Roswell Park Cancer Institute, Elm and Carlton Streets, Buffalo, NY 14263, USA

Topical photodynamic therapy (PDT) using 5-aminolevulinic acid (ALA) was approved in 1999 by the US Food and Drug Administration (FDA) for the treatment of actinic keratoses. ALA-PDT also is an effective and noninvasive treatment for several types of nonmelanoma skin cancers. Because ALA-PDT preferentially targets dysplastic, proliferating, and malignant epidermally derived and immune cells while sparing mesenchymal tissue, including dermis, multiple lesions can be treated simultaneously with rapid healing, little to no scarring, and excellent cosmetic results.

Since ALA has been readily available to investigators, it has been examined widely for skin cancers in multiple studies, as summarized in several recent reviews [1–6]. Wide variations in approach and follow-up, particularly in early work, has led to some differences in outcomes, but it is evident that ALA-PDT is an effective treatment for superficial basal cell carcinoma (sBCC) and squamous cell carcinoma (SCC) in situ. It can be useful for thin nodular basal cell carcinoma (nBCC), although it may require multiple treatments or previous tumor debulking by curettage. There also is growing evidence that it may be a valuable therapy for cutaneous malignancies other than nonmelanoma skin cancer, such as mycosis fungoides (cutaneous T-cell lymphoma; CTCL) and extramammary Paget's disease (EMPD). Because of the variable and limited depth of penetration of topical agents into the skin, ALA-PDT is not an appropriate therapy for aggressive basal cell carcinoma (BCC) subtypes (eg, morpheaform) or invasive SCC.

History

PDT has been studied since the beginning of the twentieth century [7,8], but it was not until the late 1970s that systemic PDT became a clinically relevant treatment modality. In 1978, Dr. Thomas Dougherty at Roswell Park Cancer Institute used systemic hematoporphyrin derivative, and later its partially purified form, porfimer sodium (Photofrin), to treat various malignancies effectively, including SCC and BCC [3,9]. Over the next 3 years, PDT was used worldwide to treat a variety of internal malignancies. Photofrin-PDT is useful for large or thick BCCs and for multiple nodular BCCs that may occur in the nevoid basal cell carcinoma syndrome (NBCCS) [10–12]. Photofrin-PDT is not practical for patients with limited numbers of superficial lesions, or for wide areas of thin disease on the lower legs, however, because of its cost, the possibility of dermal damage and scarring, particularly when large surface areas are treated, and the generalized cutaneous phototoxicity that is associated with systemic porfimer sodium. Photofrin-PDT also is contraindicated in children, who are more likely to develop hypertrophic scars after the procedure. In 1990, PDT became more applicable to general dermatology when Kennedy and colleagues [13] introduced

Dr. Oseroff receives ALA from DUSA, Inc. for use in investigator-designed, NIH-funded trials. Supported in part by NIH PO1-CA55791 (ARO) and by Roswell Park Cancer Institute's NCI-funded Cancer Center Support Grant CA16056.

* Corresponding author. Department of Dermatology, Roswell Park Cancer Institute, Elm and Carlton Streets, Buffalo, NY 14263.

E-mail address: allan.oseroff@roswellpark.org (A.R. Oseroff).

the use of a topical porphyrin precursor, ALA, which leads to the local accumulation of the endogenous photosensitizer protoporphyrin IX (PpIX), and which is free of prolonged cutaneous photosensitivity.

Mechanism of action

The three requirements of PDT are the presence of a photosensitizer, a light source at wavelengths that are absorbed by the photosensitizer, and oxygen. The photosensitizer preferentially accumulates in the target cells. It transfers the energy from the light source to oxygen and produces reactive oxygen species, mainly singlet oxygen [6]. PDT mediates tumor destruction in three ways: (1) production of singlet oxygen and other reactive oxygen species that damage cell membranes, mitochondria, lysosomes, and cellular microtubules, and ultimately cause direct cell death by way of necrosis and apoptosis; (2) damage to microvasculature that leads to ischemia and eventual tumor necrosis; and (3) induction of innate and adaptive immune responses, with up-regulation of inflammatory mediators (including tumor necrosis factor-α, and interleukin-1 and -6) and infiltration of neutrophils, lymphocytes, and macrophages [7,14,15]. Although important in systemic PDT, the microvasculature damage mechanism is not believed to be a significant factor in topical ALA-PDT [15,16].

5-Aminolevulinic acid and other available photosensitizers

ALA is a naturally occurring small molecule with no intrinsic photosensitizing properties that bypasses the regulatory checkpoint (ALA synthetase) in the heme synthetic pathway. If the rate of conversion of ALA to PpIX is greater than the rate of conversion of PpIX to heme, there will be transient accumulation of PpIX, the penultimate step in the pathway [5,16,17]. Malignant and premalignant carcinoma cells accumulate PpIX at a 2 to 10 fold greater rate than normal epidermis [5]. ALA-PDT selectivity is due to both structural and biochemical causes. Because ALA is a hydrophilic molecule, it is excluded by intact stratum corneum. Superficial lesions tend to have an abnormal, more permeable stratum corneum, which allows greater penetration of the ALA. Malignant and premalignant carcinoma cells accumulate PpIX at a 2 to 10 fold greater rate than normal epidermis [5]. In addition, biochemical factors,

such as lower intracellular iron (used in converting PpIX to heme) in proliferating normal malignant cells and differences in the levels of heme synthesis enzymes, contribute to the selectivity [5,17]. In the absence of light, PpIX is metabolized fully to photodynamically inactive heme over 24 to 48 hours [16]. Although circulating PpIX is the cause of photosensitivity in patients who have erythropoietic protoporphyria; with intact skin the authors have not found measurable blood levels after application of ALA under occlusion to as much as 25% of body surface area.

The Levulan Kerastick (DUSA Pharmaceuticals Inc., Wilmington, Massachusetts), a 20% solution of ALA in an alcohol-water-surfactant vehicle, along with a blue fluorescent light ($\sim$417 nm), has been approved by the FDA since 1999 for nonhyperkeratotic actinic keratoses [5,6]; it is the only commercial ALA formulation available in the United States. Pharmacy- or hospital-prepared ALA in a cream base (oil-in-water) also is used, particularly in Europe. Although the initial ALA concentration in the Kerastick is 20%, as the vehicle evaporates, the concentration increases to the limit of ALA solubility. The authors have found that under comparable conditions, the Kerastick gives higher levels of PpIX than do extemporaneous cream formulations. Occlusive dressings increase ALA penetration into the skin and increase efficacy for lesions such as BCC; they are not necessary when using for Levulan for thin actinic keratoses. The optimal application time for ALA has not been delineated clearly. Longer times allow increased penetration of ALA through the stratum corneum, and increased synthesis of PpIX. Most studies of ALA-PDT report times of 1 to 6 hours, although the authors have used 18 to 24 hours when treating large areas [18]. In their experience, overnight application of ALA under occlusion is slightly less effective than are 4- to 6-hour applications (see later discussion), but it facilitates early morning treatments in large cases [18]. For same-day application on sBCC, Morton and colleagues [19] found that 6-hour applications were more effective than 4-hour applications. It was shown that maximal surface fluorescence due to accumulated PpIX occurs at 3.5 to 5 hours for BCC and after 5 hours for actinic keratoses [20]; however, surface measurements of PpIX fluorescence may not reflect the subsurface photosensitizer levels, particularly when UV-A or blue light is used to excite the fluorescence.

The methyl ester of ALA, methyl 5-ALA (MAL), is approved in Europe for the treatment of actinic keratoses and BCCs and was approved by the FDA in 2004 for the treatment of actinic keratoses with red light [3,7]. To enter the heme synthesis pathway, MAL requires a preliminary step of conversion from MAL to ALA by way of intracellular esterases. MAL is more hydrophobic and lipophilic than is ALA, and, thus, may have greater penetration through the stratum corneum [3]. Whether these properties make MAL more efficacious than ALA in treating actinic keratoses and nonmelanoma skin cancers is unknown; a recent study showed equivalence of outcome and side effects [21].

Porfimer sodium (Photofrin) is administered systemically and results in a dose-dependent generalized cutaneous photosensitization that can last for 2 to 6 weeks [6]. It is approved by the FDA to treat Barrett's esophagus, early and late stage esophageal cancer and early-stage lung cancers. Photofrin is used off-label at half the dosage (1 mg/kg) for the treatment of nonmelanoma skin cancers with excellent outcomes [19–21]; the lower dose increases selectivity and greatly reduces cutaneous photosensitivity [21], as well as halving the cost of the drug. As noted above, its current use generally is limited to patients who have bulky or extensive dermatologic carcinomas. Verteporfin (Visudyne) is a systemically administered photosensitizer that targets blood vessels and is approved by the FDA for macular degeneration [16]. Because verteporfin only results in a few days of photosensitivity, it may have a role in treating patients who have nodular, recurrent, and multiple BCC [22], although extensive vascular damage may cause significant scarring.

Light sources

ALA-induced PpIX, which has a peak absorption in the Soret band ($\sim$410 nm), with four much smaller peaks near 510 nm, 540 nm, 580 nm, and 635 nm [23]. Because of this wide range, multiple light sources with different spectral outputs can be used in PDT [5]; however, the relevant parameter in PDT is the dose of absorbed light, rather than what is delivered. For example, the DUSA Blu-U fluorescent light with a wavelength of 417 ± 5 nm and an irradiance of 10 mW/cm^2 is absorbed about 20-fold more strongly than is light at 635 nm. Therefore, a 10 J/cm^2 Blu-U light dose can be equivalent to as much as 200 J/cm^2 red light at 635 nm. Conversely, white light from a tungsten halogen source ($\sim$410–730 nm) is inefficient, because much of its output is at wavelengths not absorbed by PpIX. Similarly, red light from a narrow band filtered lamp, such as the Patterson PDT light (630 nm $\pm$ 15 nm) (Photo Therapeutics, Inc., Altrincham, Cheshire, England) that was used by Morton and colleagues [24] or from a 633-nm light emitting diode (LED) array, is absorbed more efficiently than is the 580-nm to 750-nm output from more broadly filtered lamps, such as the Waldmann PDT 1200 L (Waldmann Medizintechnik/FRG). A recent study showed that 40 J/cm^2 from an LED array was clinically equivalent to 100 J/cm^2 from the PDT 1200 L [25]. Note that PpIX irradiation causes formation of a photoproduct absorbing near 670 nm that can be activated by the broadly filtered red lamps, which may contribute to their clinical efficacy.

When choosing a wavelength, the depth of penetration also needs to be considered. Tissue penetration increases with wavelength, because of decreasing tissue scattering and decreased absorption by hemoglobin and melanin. In particular, hemoglobin absorption bands overlap those of PpIX at wavelengths less than 600 nm. The most strongly absorbed photosensitizing wavelength, approximately 410 nm, penetrates only 1 to 2 mm in skin, whereas 635-nm red light penetrates up to 6 mm [16]. The lack of penetration of blue fluorescent lights makes them more suitable for treating superficial lesions, such as actinic keratoses [2]. Blue light also might be effective for Bowen's disease, although it might be expected to miss disease that extends down into skin appendages. Most investigators believe that red light is preferable for treating skin cancer because it takes advantage of the absorption peak at 635 nm while maximizing penetration [7].

Light sources that are used for PDT include lasers, xenon arc and incandescent filament lamps, and light-emitting diodes [16]. Because no single light source has been shown to be ideal for ALA-PDT, the choice depends on the clinical indications, and the desired field-size, treatment time, and cost [2]. Tungsten-halogen–based, broad-spectrum noncoherent light sources are used more extensively than are lasers because of reduced cost, increased safety, and portability [7]. Recently, Clark and colleagues [26] reported similar efficacy for broadband and laser light sources when using ALA-PDT to treat actinic keratoses, superficial BCC, and Bowen's disease. After treating Bowen's disease with ALA-PDT using a pulsed dye laser (585 nm, 7 J/cm^2), Britton and colleagues [27] concluded that lasers were tolerated better and reduced exposure time; however, they required more operator skill than did noncoherent light sources. Treatment-associated pain scales with illuminated surface area, so that sources, such as the pulsed dye laser or intense pulsed light sources that sequentially illuminate small areas, may have advantages, along with higher costs.

In summary, when treating skin cancers with ALA-PDT, the ideal light source, wavelength, irradiance, and total dosage of light have not been established firmly; however, some generalizations can be made. Light with a wavelength near 635 nm is likely the most effective in the treatment of skin cancers for the reasons that were discussed above. When using nonlaser red light sources, light doses of 100 to 150 J/cm^2 are appropriate [6,18]. Using a laser source, the carcinoma response with fluence seems to follow a sigmoidal pattern, with a rapidly increasing response with light dose leading to a "knee" in the response curve around 100 to 150 J/cm^2, when the response rate approaches 90% [18]; doses of 200 J/cm^2 give high initial response rates. When treating skin cancers, the irradiance or light intensity usually has ranged between 40 and 150 mW/cm^2, and it should not exceed 200 mW/cm^2 to avoid hyperthermic injury [2,6,7].

Basal cell carcinoma

ALA-PDT is a useful treatment for superficial BCC. A review by the British Photodermatology Group concluded that there was strong evidence for efficacy [2], and topical PDT is used routinely for sBCC in Europe. A wide range in reported results reflects the multiplicity of approaches taken by different investigators, including significant differences in light doses, as well as large variations in follow-up times [1,2,5]. Some of the many results are summarized in Table 1. In 1990, Kennedy and colleagues [13] were the first to report the treatment of sBCC with ALA-PDT (3- to 6-hour application of ALA followed by filtered red light, 600+ nm); 300 cases of sBCC were treated with a 79% clearance rate at 3 months. More recently, Morton and colleagues [24] used ALA-PDT to treat 98 large or multiple superficial BCCs and noted an 89% clearance rate after one or more treatments; it was suggested by the investigators that ALA-PDT might be superior to electrosurgery for large BCC and excision for multiple BCC. Clark and colleagues [26] reported a 97% (84/87) clearance rate for superficial BCC that was treated monthly up to four times with ALA applied for 6 hours followed by one of three similar red lamps (~570–720 nm), or a 630-nm diode laser; the light dose was about 125 J/cm^2. The number of required treatments increased with lesion diameter. The recurrence rate was 4.8% with a median follow-up of 55 weeks. Wang and colleagues [28] compared ALA-PDT with cryotherapy (6-hour application of ALA followed by a 635-nm dye laser; 60 J/cm^2) for the treatment of superficial and nodular BCC. Lesions were followed clinically and biopsied at 3 months; they were retreated on clinical grounds or for histopathologic tumor, and biopsied again at 12 months. Thirty percent of the PDT lesions

Table 1
Studies examining aminolevulinic acid photodynamic therapy for superficial basal cell carcinoma

Study	Number of tumors treated	Complete clearance rate	Recurrence rate (Follow-up)	Light source
Kennedy et al [13]	300	79%	–	Red light (600 + nm)
Clark et al [26]	87	97%	4.8% (55 wk)	Red light or 630-nm laser
Wang et al [28]	21	100%	5% clinically 38% by histology (12 mo)	635-nm laser
Morton et al [56]	98	89%	7% (34–41 mo)	Red light (630 ± 15 nm)
Haller et al [30]	26	100% 2 treatments	4% (27 mo)	Red light (630 ± 15 nm)
Oseroff et al (unpublished data)	95 (4–6 h ALA) 98 (18–24 h ALA)	99% (4–6 h ALA) 94% (18–24 h ALA)	1% (12 mo) 14% (36 mo)	633-nm laser ≥ 200 J/cm^2

needed retreatments. The investigators noted no significant difference in efficacy between PDT and cryotherapy, but the group that was treated with ALA-PDT noted fewer adverse events, faster healing times, and better cosmetic results. At 12 months, 5% of the PDT-treated BCCs were clinical failures, but an additional 20% of the treatment sites that were clinically clear had residual BCC on biopsy. Therefore, short-term clinical follow-up may give misleadingly high response rates.

In an ongoing study, the authors have used topical 20% ALA in a cream base applied under occlusion for either 4 to 6 hours or 18 to 24 hours. Using single treatments with 633-nm laser irradiation at high light doses (200–300 J/cm^2 at 150 mW/cm^2), they found complete clinical responses in 94 of 95 (99%) sBCCs with 4- to 6-hour ALA, and in 93 of 98 (94%) sBCCs with 18- to 24-hour ALA assessed 6 months after PDT (unpublished data). There was no improvement going from 200 to 300 J/cm^2, which is consistent with the sigmoidal shape of the response versus light dose curve [18]. Follow-up ranged from 16 months to more than 72 months. Recurrence rates were about 14% at 3 years, and retreatment of recurrences had about the same efficacy as did initial treatments (unpublished data). The single-treatment response results are higher than those reported by other investigators (see Table 1), possibly because of the higher light doses.

ALA-PDT is less effective for nBCC. In a review of 12 early studies by Peng and colleagues [1], the complete clearance rate of 826 sBCCs and 208 nBCCs was 87% and 53%, respectively; more recent reports give clearance rates of only 10% to 75% [5]. In the authors' ongoing trial, they obtained complete clinical responses 6 months after PDT in 44 of 51 (86%) biopsy-proven nBCCs using single treatments without skin preparation, but with light doses of 200 J/cm^2 (unpublished data).

Is red light necessary? Morton and colleagues [23] compared red light (630 ± 15 nm) with green light (540 ± 15 nm). They found that the latter was substantially worse, with initial and 12-month complete response rates of 72% and 48%, respectively, compared with 94% and 88%, respectively, for red illumination. Similarly, the overall efficacy of 417 nm blue light generally appears lower. In a preliminary study, the Blu-U lamp was used with multiple sessions of ALA-PDT (ALA applied for 1 to 5 hours) to treat 2 patients with NBCCS [37]. The complete clinical response rates for sBCC were better on the face than the lower extremities (8 of 9 [89%] vs 18 of 27 [67%], respectively) with only 8 month follow ups, and response rates were much lower for nBCC on the face (5 of 16 [31%]). While treatment conditions might not have been optimal, the blue light response rates were substantially worse than what have been reported with red light (see Table 1). Thus, red light is preferable for carcinomas.

Even with red light, ALA-PDT's lower effectiveness in treating nBCC may be due to inadequate penetration of ALA into the deeper portions of the skin and the malignancy [5], but it also might reflect biologic heterogeneity in accumulation of PpIX within the carcinoma. The authors and colleagues have found that although PpIX fluorescence extended to the base of lesions that were 3- to 5-mm thick, there was inconsistent accumulation of PpIX within nBCC (unpublished data). In addition, follow-up histology showed PDT effects within the dermis at depths greater than the thickness of original carcinomas [29], which suggests that PpIX had penetrated through the lesions.

Several strategies have been studied to enhance effectiveness. One approach is to repeat PDT routinely. Haller and colleagues [30] treated 26 sBCCs with two sessions of ALA-PDT (ALA applied for 4 hours followed by nonlaser light of 630 ± 15 nm, 50 to 100 mW/cm^2, 120 to 134 J/cm^2) 1 week apart; the investigators reported a 100% response rate and a recurrence rate of only 4% at 27 months of follow-up. This is not surprising, because if the efficacy of the repetitive treatment was simply additive, a single-treatment response rate of 80% or 90% would increase to 96% or 98%, respectively, with two treatments; both are within the confidence interval surrounding a 100% response rate with only 26 lesions. A drawback of routine double treatments is the increased cost. Another approach is to debulk the BCC before PDT. Thissen and colleagues [31] reported a clearance rate of 92% (22 of 24) for nBCC after a single cycle of ALA-PDT (noncoherent red light, 100 mW/cm^2, 120 J/cm^2), when preceded by a curettage debulking 3 weeks earlier. Again, this improvement is not unexpected because curettage alone is an effective treatment for BCC [32], and placebo studies with MAL-PDT show that even mild debulking by itself gives as much as a 20% complete response rate. A third approach attempts to increase the ALA within the BCC. Iontophoresis and the addition of dimethyl sulfoxide (DMSO) or EDTA have been used in an attempt to increase the penetration and effects of

ALA [33,34]. Intralesional ALA administration has been proposed for nBCC, but there are no comparative data that demonstrate increased efficacy [35,36].

ALA-PDT may be particularly useful in certain clinical situations. For example, it may be a valuable adjuvant treatment for extensive BCC. Kuijpers and colleagues [37] used ALA-PDT in four patients after Mohs surgery; they reported complete remission and excellent clinical and cosmetic results for a follow-up period of 27 months. Also, ALA-PDT was useful in the treatment of patients with NBCCS [15,38].

In summary, ALA-PDT is suited ideally for patients who have multiple, or large superficial BCC [2], and for sites where minimal dermal injury (eg, lower legs) and excellent cosmetic outcome are a priority. The authors' results suggest that high light doses improve outcome, but also increase treatment time and discomfort. Under currently used treatment conditions, ALA-PDT is less effective for nBCC, and may require debulking or multiple treatments. PDT also may have value as an adjunct to traditional therapy (eg, Mohs surgery). Morpheaform and other aggressive forms of BCC and lesions without clinically defined borders should not be treated with ALA-PDT.

Bowen's disease

ALA-PDT is an excellent treatment for Bowen's disease (SCC in situ), and it should be considered in patients who have large or multiple lesions, or lesions on poor healing areas (eg, lower legs), and areas that are less amenable to traditional treatment (eg, face or genitals) (Table 2) [7,16]. Successful treatment of Bowen's disease was described first in 1990 by Kennedy and colleagues [13]; they reported the complete clearance of SCC in situ in six patients (3- to 6-hour application of ALA followed by red light). In 2002, Morton and colleagues [2] reviewed the available literature on ALA-PDT for Bowen's disease and reported an 86% clearance rate after only a single treatment, a 93% clearance rate with one or two repeat treatments, and an average recurrence rate of 12% up to 36 months after treatment. Using 200 J/cm^2 light doses, the authors obtained complete clinical responses in 92% (23/25) of lesions with 4- to 6-hour ALA application; the complete response rate was 81% (21/26) with 18- to 24-hour ALA application (unpublished data). Although the longer application time has a trend toward a lower clearance rate, the differences are not statistically significant.

ALA-PDT has comparable or better efficacy than does cryotherapy or topical 5-fluouracil (5-FU), with fewer adverse events and superior cosmetic results. Morton and colleagues [39] treated 40 biopsy-proven SCC in situ lesions that were less than 2 cm diameter with cryotherapy or ALA-PDT (ALA applied for 4 hours followed by red light, 70 mW/cm^2, 125 J/cm^2). Although only 50% of the lesions that were treated with cryotherapy cleared, there was

Table 2
Studies examining aminolevulinic acid photodynamic therapy for Bowen's Disease

Study	Number of tumors treated	Complete clearance rate	Recurrence rate (Follow-up)	Light source
Kennedy et al [13]	6	100%	–	Red light (600 + nm)
Morton et al [39]	20	75% (100% after 2nd treatment)	0% (12 mo)	Red light (630 ± 15 nm)
Morton et al [56]	32	94%	7% (12 mo)	Red light (630 ± 15 nm)
Morton et al [56]	29	72%	33% (12 mo)	Green light (540 ± 15 nm)
Salim et al [40]	33	88%	7% (12 mo)	Red light (630 ± 15 nm)
Clark et al [26]	129	91%	10.3% (44 wk)	Red light or 630-nm laser
Britton et al [27]	17	82%	0% (12 mo)	585-nm pulsed dye laser
Oseroff et al (unpublished data)	25 (4–6 h ALA) 26 (18–24 h ALA)	92% (4–6 h ALA) 81% (18–24 h ALA)	6% (24 mo)	633-nm laser 200 J/cm^2

a 75% and 100% clearance rate after one and two sessions of PDT, respectively. Although the differences between PDT and cryotherapy were not statistically significant, the study showed that ALA-PDT is an effective treatment option for Bowen's disease. A later study by Salim and colleagues [40] demonstrated that ALA-PDT is more effective for Bowen's disease than topical 5-FU, and it should be considered a first-line therapy. Forty patients who had Bowen's disease were randomized to 5-FU or ALA-PDT (ALA applied for 4 hours followed by narrowband red light, 630 ± 15 nm, 50–90 mW/cm^2, 100 J/cm^2); the group that underwent ALA-PDT had an 88% clearance rate as compared with 67% in the group that received 5-FU.

Britton and colleagues [27] employed a pulsed dye laser (585 nm) with ALA-PDT for the treatment of 17 patches of Bowen's disease; the results were comparable to other studies that used non-laser light sources, with 82% complete clinical response. Clark and colleagues [26] reported a 91% (117/129) clearance rate for Bowen's disease with a 10.3% recurrence rate at 44 weeks (ALA applied for 4 hours followed by red light lamps or a 630 nm diode laser). Finally, Morton and colleagues [23] investigated the efficacy of using red (630 ± 15 nm, 86 mW/cm^2, 125 J/cm^2) versus green (540 ± 15 nm, 86 mW/cm^2, 62.5 J/cm^2) light for ALA-PDT for Bowen's disease; the red light was superior in obtaining a 94% (88% at 12 months) clearance rate as compared with 72% (48% at 12 months) for the green light.

Although ALA-PDT is an excellent treatment for SCC in situ, with the treatment conditions that have been examined, it is not indicated for invasive SCC because of poor initial response rates and unacceptable high recurrence rates [16]. In patients who have a mixture of actinic keratoses and Bowen's disease, it is important to biopsy lesions that persist after PDT, because they may be invasive SCC [41].

Treatment of cutaneous malignancies other than nonmelanoma skin cancers

Mycosis fungoides, a type of CTCL, is the most common type of cutaneous lymphoma [42]. The treatment of mycosis fungoides can be challenging and there is no treatment that has shown to increase overall survival. Although the literature is mostly anecdotal, there is evidence that ALA-PDT may be a viable treatment option for localized disease [43–46]. The authors have found

application of ALA solution under occlusion for 4 hours, followed by irradiation with a 595-nm long pulse dye laser, to be effective in eradicating localized infiltrates in a patient receiving photopheresis, and it was superior to topical steroids. In addition, other cutaneous lymphomas, including CD8$^+$ CTCL, anaplastic large cell lymphoma, and cutaneous B-cell lymphoma, have been treated successfully with ALA-PDT [43,47,48]. Although the current reports are promising, more studies need to be done before ALA-PDT becomes a standard treatment for cutaneous lymphomas.

EMPD is a rare, multifocal intraepithelial malignancy that presents commonly as well-demarcated, pruritic plaques in apocrine-bearing regions of older adults; it often recurs after surgery, even when clear margins were obtained [49]. Shieh and colleagues [49] reported the results of 16 cases of EMPD treated with ALA-PDT and systemic Photofrin-PDT. The clearance rates were comparable to standard surgical treatment, but without the scarring and associated morbidity of surgery. Given the frequent local recurrence and problems that are associated with extensive surgery, treatment with ALA-PDT may be justified, even if the complete response rate does not reach the levels that are obtained for sBCC and Bowen's disease [50].

Cancer detection and prevention

ALA-PDT may have a role in cancer detection in patients who undergo transplant and other high-risk patients [5]. Because precancerous and cancerous cells have an increased uptake of ALA, there is a significantly increased amount of fluorescence when compared with normal surrounding skin. This fluorescence may be able to help clinicians outline tumor margins and detect early subclinical or recurrent disease [51]. A potential problem is that PpIX also accumulates in sites of inflammation, so false positives are possible.

Theoretically, PDT also could be used in high-risk patients to destroy premalignant cells selectively and prevent the future development of skin cancers. ALA-PDT delayed photocarcinogenesis in mice [52,53], and there is a suggestion that it may prevent the development of skin cancer in high-risk, NBCCS patients [18]. This idea was tested in immunosuppressed patients by de Graff and colleagues [54], who treated 40 organ transplant recipients with ALA-PDT; however, they did not detect a significant decrease in the development of SCC within a 2-year follow-up period. Because their treatment conditions had no effect on existing disease it is difficult to interpret their findings. In contrast, a study by Dragieva and colleagues [55] of ALA-PDT for actinic keratoses and Bowen's disease in transplant recipients using more aggressive treatment had an initial response of 88%, compared with 94% in immunocompetent controls. Residual subclinical disease remained, however, because the immunosuppressed patients had a 20% recurrence rate at 12 weeks and a 40% recurrence rate at 48 weeks, far higher than in the immunocompetent controls [55]. It is possible immune and inflammatory processes eliminated the subclinical residual in the immunocompetent patients.

PDT can act as a biologic response modifier by stimulating innate and adaptive immune responses and possibly by generating anti-tumor vaccines [15]. The fact that some patients who undergo PDT seem to get fewer additional skin cancers may be due to the destruction of subclinical lesions, or to induction of an antitumor response that suppresses development of new carcinomas [15,18]. If the latter is true, this may explain, at least in part, the above findings by Dragieva and colleagues [55].

Safety and side effect profile

Generally, ALA-PDT is tolerated well with only transient side effects reported [5]. Discomfort is the most common problem; patients often complain of burning, pruritus, and stinging during PDT and for a few hours afterwards [6]. Pain increases with treated surface area. Therefore, ALA-PDT for diffuse actinic keratoses may result in greater discomfort than for BCC or SCC in situ, likely because of the adjacent subclinical disease that also gets treated [16]. The pain can be relieved with administration of analgesics, use of cooling fans, and spraying water on lesions during treatment. Large-area, aggressive therapy may warrant conscious sedation or monitored anesthesia care. ALA is unstable at neutral or basic pH. Thus, application of topical anesthetics that have a pH of 7 or greater should be avoided because it may result in the inactivation of the ALA, especially if the anesthetic application overlaps short ALA application times. EMLA is particularly problematic, because it has a pH of 9.

The patient may experience local photosensitivity for a few hours after the treatment, so proper clothing and sun avoidance are necessary after treatment. The skin should be cleaned with water to remove any surface ALA that subsequently might be converted to PpIX. After ALA-PDT, erythema and edema, followed by erosion and crust formation, are expected, with complete healing within 2 to 6 weeks [16]. Rarely, patients may experience postinflammatory hypopigmentation and hyperpigmentation; changes usually are transient and more prevalent in darker skin.

PpIX does not accumulate in the cell's nucleus, and singlet oxygen has a short diffusion distance within the cell; however, ALA-PDT has potential mutagenic effects and has been shown to produce DNA strand breaks, chromosomal aberrations, and alkylation of DNA [2,16]. In addition, topical PDT has a low risk for acting as a tumor-promoting agent [5]. Although the risk for carcinogenesis probably is extremely small, long-term monitoring is warranted, given the lengthy latent period for carcinogenesis [2].

Summary

ALA-PDT is an effective and noninvasive therapy for sBCC and Bowen's disease. It also may have a role in the treatment of nBCC and other cutaneous malignancies, including localized cutaneous lymphomas. ALA-PDT offers multiple advantages over traditional treatments, including little to no scarring, excellent cosmetic results, and the ability to treat multiple lesions simultaneously; however, it is not an effective therapy for invasive SCC or aggressive subtypes of BCC. Finally, ALA-PDT may be a useful way to prevent new skin cancers in certain high-risk patients.

References

[1] Peng Q, Warloe T, Berg K, et al. 5-Aminolevulinic acid-based photodynamic therapy. Clinical research and future challenges. Cancer 1997;79(12):2282–308.
[2] Morton C, Brown S, Collins S, et al. Guidelines for topical photodynamic therapy: report of a workshop of the British Photodermatology Group. Br J Derm 2002;146:552–67.
[3] Zeitouni NC, Oseroff AR, Shieh S. Photodynamic therapy for nonmelanoma skin cancers. Current review and update. Mol Immunol 2003;39(17–18):1133–6.
[4] Marmur ES, Schmults CD, Goldberg DJ. A review of laser and photodynamic therapy for the treatment of nonmelanoma skin cancer. Dermatol Surg 2004;30(2 Pt 2):264–71.

[5] Kormeili T, Yamauchi PS, Lowe NJ. Topical photo-dynamic therapy in clinical dermatology. Br J Dermatol 2004;150(6):1061–9.

[6] Babilas P, Karrer S, Sidoroff A, et al. Photodynamic therapy in dermatology–an update. Photodermatol Photoimmunol Photomed 2005;21(3):142–9.

[7] Garcia-Zuazaga J, Cooper KD, Baron ED. Photodynamic therapy in dermatology: current concepts in the treatment of skin cancer. Expert Rev Anticancer Ther 2005;5(5):791–800.

[8] Daniell MD, Hill JS. A history of photodynamic therapy. Aust N Z J Surg 1991;61(5):340–8.

[9] Dougherty TJ. A brief history of clinical photodynamic therapy development at Roswell Park Cancer Institute. J Clin Laser Med Surg 1996;14(5):219–21.

[10] Wilson BD, Mang TS, Stoll H, et al. Photodynamic therapy for the treatment of basal cell carcinoma. Arch Dermatol 1992;128(12):1597–601.

[11] Jones CM, Mang T, Cooper M, et al. Photodynamic therapy in the treatment of Bowen's disease. J Am Acad Dermatol 1992;27:979–82.

[12] Oseroff AR, Blumenson LE, Wilson BD, et al. A dose ranging study of photodynamic therapy with porfimer sodium (Photofrin?) for treatment of basal cell carcinoma. Lasers Med Sci 2006;38(5):417–26.

[13] Kennedy JC, Pottier RH, Pross DC. Photodynamic therapy with endogenous protoporphyrin IX: basic principles and present clinical experience. J Photochem Photobiol B 1990;6(1–2):143–8.

[14] Gollnick SO, Liu X, Owczarczak B, et al. Altered expression of interleukin 6 and interleukin 10 as a result of photodynamic therapy in vivo. Cancer Res 1997;57(18):3904–9.

[15] Oseroff AR. PDT as a cytotoxic agent and biological response modifier: implications for cancer prevention and treatment in immunosuppressed and immunocompetent patients. J Invest Dermatol 2006;126(3):542–4.

[16] Morton CA. Photodynamic therapy for nonmelanoma skin cancer–and more? Arch Dermatol 2004;140(1):116–20.

[17] Rittenhouse-Diakun K, van Leengoed H, Morgan J, et al. The role of transferrin receptor (CD71) in photodynamic therapy of activated and malignant lymphocytes using the heme precursor delta-aminolevulinic acid (ALA). Photochem Photobiol 1995;61(5):523–8.

[18] Oseroff AR, Shieh S, Frawley NP, et al. Treatment of diffuse basal cell carcinomas and basaloid follicular hamartomas in nevoid basal cell carcinoma syndrome by wide-area 5-aminolevulinic acid photodynamic therapy. Arch Dermatol 2005;141(1):60–7.

[19] Morton CA, MacKie RM, Whitehurst C, et al. Photodynamic therapy for basal cell carcinoma: effect of tumor thickness and duration of photosensitizer application on response. Arch Dermatol 1998;134(2):248–9.

[20] Stefanidou M, Tosca A, Themelis G, et al. In vivo fluorescence kinetics and photodynamic therapy efficacy of delta-aminolevulinic acid-induced porphyrins in basal cell carcinomas and actinic keratoses; implications for optimization of photodynamic therapy. Eur J Dermatol 2000;10(5):351–6.

[21] Kuijpers DI, Thissen MR, Thissen CA, et al. Similar effectiveness of methyl aminolevulinate and 5-aminolevulinate in topical photodynamic therapy for nodular basal cell carcinoma. J Drugs Dermatol 2006;5(7):642–5.

[22] Lui H, Hobbs L, Tope WD, et al. Photodynamic therapy of multiple nonmelanoma skin cancers with verteporfin and red light-emitting diodes: two-year results evaluating tumor response and cosmetic outcomes. Arch Dermatol 2004;140(1):26–32.

[23] Morton CA, Whitehurst C, Moore JV, et al. Comparison of red and green light in the treatment of Bowen's disease by photodynamic therapy. Br J Dermatol 2000;143(4):767–72.

[24] Morton CA, Whitehurst C, McColl JH, et al. Photodynamic therapy for large or multiple patches of Bowen disease and basal cell carcinoma. Arch Dermatol 2001;137(3):319–24.

[25] Babilas P, Kohl E, Maisch T, et al. In vitro and in vivo comparison of two different light sources for topical photodynamic therapy. Br J Dermatol 2006;154(4):712–8.

[26] Clark C, Bryden A, Dawe R, et al. Topical 5-aminolaevulinic acid photodynamic therapy for cutaneous lesions: outcome and comparison of light sources. Photodermatol Photoimmunol Photomed 2003;19(3):134–41.

[27] Britton JE, Goulden V, Stables G, et al. Investigation of the use of the pulsed dye laser in the treatment of Bowen's disease using 5-aminolaevulinic acid phototherapy. Br J Dermatol 2005;153(4):780–4.

[28] Wang I, Bendsoe N, Klinteberg CA, et al. Photodynamic therapy vs. cryosurgery of basal cell carcinomas: results of a phase III clinical trial. Br J Dermatol 2001;144(4):832–40.

[29] Fink-Puches R, Soyer HP, Hofer A, et al. Long-term follow-up and histological changes of superficial nonmelanoma skin cancers treated with topical delta-aminolevulinic acid photodynamic therapy. Arch Dermatol 1998;134(7):821–6.

[30] Haller JC, Cairnduff F, Slack G, et al. Routine double treatments of superficial basal cell carcinomas using aminolaevulinic acid-based photodynamic therapy. Br J Dermatol 2000;143(6):1270–5.

[31] Thissen MR, Schroeter CA, Neumann HA. Photodynamic therapy with delta-aminolaevulinic acid for nodular basal cell carcinomas using a prior debulking technique. Br J Dermatol 2000;142(2):338–9.

[32] Barlow JO, Zalla MJ, Kyle A, et al. Treatment of basal cell carcinoma with curettage alone. J Am Acad Dermatol 2006;54(6):1039–45.

[33] Rhodes LE, Tsoukas MM, Anderson RR, et al. Iontophoretic delivery of ALA provides a quantitative model for ALA pharmacokinetics and PpIX phototoxicity in human skin. J Invest Dermatol 1997; 108(1):87–91.

[34] Choudry K, Brooke RC, Farrar W, et al. The effect of an iron chelating agent on protoporphyrin IX levels and phototoxicity in topical 5-aminolaevulinic acid photodynamic therapy. Br J Dermatol 2003; 149(1):124–30.

[35] Cappugi P, Mavilia L, Campolmi P, et al. New proposal for the treatment of nodular basal cell carcinoma with intralesional 5-aminolevulinic acid. J Chemother 2004;16(5):491–3.

[36] de Blois AW, Grouls RJ, Ackerman EW, et al. Development of a stable solution of 5-aminolaevulinic acid for intracutaneous injection in photodynamic therapy. Lasers Med Sci 2002;17(3):208–15.

[37] Kuijpers DI, Smeets NW, Krekels GA, et al. Photodynamic therapy as adjuvant treatment of extensive basal cell carcinoma treated with Mohs micrographic surgery. Dermatol Surg 2004;30(5): 794–8.

[38] Itkin A, Gilchrest BA. Delta-Aminolevulinic acid and blue light photodynamic therapy for treatment of multiple basal cell carcinomas in two patients with nevoid basal cell carcinoma syndrome. Dermatol Surg 2004;30(7):1054–61.

[39] Morton CA, Whitehurst C, Moseley H, et al. Comparison of photodynamic therapy with cryotherapy in the treatment of Bowen's disease. Br J Dermatol 1996;135(5):766–71.

[40] Salim A, Leman JA, McColl JH, et al. Randomized comparison of photodynamic therapy with topical 5-fluorouracil in Bowen's disease. Br J Dermatol 2003;148(3):539–43.

[41] Alexiades-Armenakas MR, Geronemus RG. Laser-mediated photodynamic therapy of actinic keratoses. Arch Dermatol 2003;139(10):1313–20.

[42] Girardi M, Heald PW, Wilson LD. The pathogenesis of mycosis fungoides. N Engl J Med 2004; 350(19):1978–88.

[43] Coors EA, von den Driesch P. Topical photodynamic therapy for patients with therapy-resistant lesions of cutaneous T-cell lymphoma. J Am Acad Dermatol 2004;50(3):363–7.

[44] Edstrom DW, Porwit A, Ros AM. Photodynamic therapy with topical 5-aminolevulinic acid for mycosis fungoides: clinical and histological response. Acta Derm Venereol 2001;81(3):184–8.

[45] Orenstein A, Haik J, Tamir J, et al. Photodynamic therapy of cutaneous lymphoma using 5-aminolevulinic acid topical application. Dermatol Surg 2000; 26(8):765–9.

[46] Markham T, Sheahan K, Collins P. Topical 5-aminolaevulinic acid photodynamic therapy for tumour-stage mycosis fungoides. Br J Dermatol 2001; 144(6):1262–3.

[47] Mori M, Campolmi P, Mavilia L, et al. Topical photodynamic therapy for primary cutaneous B-cell lymphoma: a pilot study. J Am Acad Dermatol 2006; 54(3):524–6.

[48] Umegaki N, Moritsugu R, Katoh S, et al. Photodynamic therapy may be useful in debulking cutaneous lymphoma prior to radiotherapy. Clin Exp Dermatol 2004;29(1):42–5.

[49] Shieh S, Dee AS, Cheney RT, et al. Photodynamic therapy for the treatment of extramammary Paget's disease. Br J Dermatol 2002;146(6):1000–5.

[50] Tulchinsky H, Zmora O, Brazowski E, et al. Extramammary Paget's disease of the perianal region. Colorectal Dis 2004;6(3):206–9.

[51] Fritsch C, Lang K, Neuse W, et al. Photodynamic diagnosis and therapy in dermatology. Skin Pharmacol Appl Skin Physiol 1998;11(6):358–73.

[52] Stender IM, Bech-Thomsen N, Poulsen T, et al. Photodynamic therapy with topical delta-aminolevulinic acid delays UV photocarcinogenesis in hairless mice. Photochem Photobiol 1997;66(4):493–6.

[53] Sharfaei S, Viau G, Lui H, et al. Systemic photodynamic therapy with aminolaevulinic acid delays the appearance of ultraviolet-induced skin tumours in mice. Br J Dermatol 2001;144(6):1207–14.

[54] de Graaf YG, Kennedy C, Wolterbeek R, et al. Photodynamic therapy does not prevent cutaneous squamous-cell carcinoma in organ-transplant recipients: results of a randomized-controlled trial. J Invest Dermatol 2006;126(3):569–74.

[55] Dragieva G, Hafner J, Dummer R, et al. Topical photodynamic therapy in the treatment of actinic keratoses and Bowen's disease in transplant recipients. Transplantation 2004;77(1):115–21.

[56] Morton C, Whitehurst C, McColl JH, et al. Photodynamic therapy for large or multiple patches of Bowen Disease and basal cell carcinoma. Arch Dermatol 2001;137:319–24.

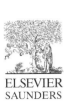

ELSEVIER
SAUNDERS

Dermatol Clin 25 (2007) 15–23

Photodynamic Therapy for Actinic Keratoses

Michal S. Kalisiak, MD, Jaggi Rao, MD, FRCPC*

*Division of Dermatology and Cutaneous Sciences, University of Alberta, 2-125 Clinical Sciences Building,
Edmonton, Alberta T6G 2G3, Canada*

Actinic keratoses (AKs) are one of the most common conditions that are treated by dermatologists; they account for 14% of dermatology office visits in the United States [1]. The exact prevalence varies widely, depending on the population studied and geographic latitude, and reaches more than 40% in the general population in some studies. Risk factors for development of AKs include UV exposure, fair skin (skin types I–III), advancing age, and immunosuppression [2].

The rationale for treating AKs stems from their potential to evolve into invasive squamous cell carcinoma (SCC), which is estimated to occur in about 8% of cases [3]. Because SCC can metastasize and prove fatal, treatment of AKs provides a window of opportunity in the prevention of invasive cancer. Traditionally, treatment options were based on physical destruction, topical chemotherapy, and, more recently, application of immune response modifiers. From the 1990s, photodynamic therapy (PDT) has been included in this armamentarium as a novel, versatile method for treating AKs [4,5].

This article focuses on the use of 5-aminolevulinic acid photodynamic therapy (ALA-PDT) and methyl aminolevulinate (MAL) PDT for the treatment of AKs. The key to successful PDT is to understand the physicochemical basis of this technique and how this relates to patient and lesion characteristics. Practical application requires knowledge of photosensitizers and activating light sources. Numerous trials that documented efficacy are reviewed. Finally, specific PDT techniques are outlined and various pitfalls are presented.

Clinical and histopathologic aspects of actinic keratoses

AKs usually are diagnosed clinically based on their appearance of scaly, erythematous papules and plaques that are found on sun-damaged skin, predominantly on the scalp, face, dorsal hands, and lower extremities. Variant lesions may be hyperkeratotic (including those that present with a cutaneous horn) AKs or pigmented AKs. Most often they are asymptomatic, but may cause burning, pruritus, tenderness, or bleeding. Actinic cheilitis, which occurs most commonly on the sun-exposed lower lip, represents a subtype of AKs with particular tendency to progress to SCC [5,6].

The histopathology of AKs is characterized by proliferation of atypical keratinocytes in architecturally abnormal epidermis. Cytologic features, which are indistinguishable from those seen in SCC, include loss of polarity, nuclear pleomorphism, disordered maturation, and an increased number of mitotic figures that may be atypical. Architectural distortion is exemplified by focal parakeratosis, underlying hypogranulosis, irregular acanthosis, and presence of small downward-oriented buds at the basal layer. Invariably, there is an underlying solar elastosis, and, often, a mild chronic inflammatory cell infiltrate. Protrusion of atypical keratinocytes and their nests into the dermis is the hallmark of malignant degeneration to invasive SCC. Often, the differentiation between AKs and SCC in situ (Bowen's disease) is a matter of judgment [7]. As such, AKs are considered widely to be in a continuum with SCC. The term "keratinocytic intraepidermal neoplasia" has been coined for this continuum, in analogy to

Drs. M. Kalisiak and J. Rao have no financial conflicts and received no honoraria in conjunction with this work.

* Corresponding author.
E-mail address: jrao@ualberta.ca (J. Rao).

doi:10.1016/j.det.2006.09.006

"cervical intraepithelial neoplasia" that is used in gynecology [2,6]. Inclusion of AKs on this spectrum lends further urgency to provision of reliable treatment.

Traditional approaches to treatment of actinic keratoses

Numerous treatment options exist for AKs, including cryosurgery, curettage, excision, dermabrasion, chemical peels, laser resurfacing, 5-fluorouracil (5-FU), topical diclofenac, topical retinoids, and topical immune response modifiers (eg, imiquimod). Each of these methods has a unique set of characteristics and may be considered advantageous in certain circumstances. Clinical parameters that impact therapeutic choice include thickness of the lesions, quantity, anatomic location, skin type, patient preferences, cost, reimbursement options, desire for cosmesis, availability of equipment and training, and the practitioner's familiarity with the therapeutic intervention [5]. PDT offers a versatile technique in which parameters can be varied to suit diverse clinical situations [5,8,9].

Physicochemical basis of photodynamic therapy

PDT begins with application of the porphyrin precursor, 5-ALA, or its derivative, MAL, to the skin, its penetration to target cells, and its rapid in situ conversion to photosensitive protoporphyrin IX (PpIX). The newly synthesized PpIX accumulates inside cells and is activated by delivery of light to the treated tissue. Photoactivation of PpIX results in production of toxic singlet oxygen and other cytotoxic free radicals that lead to tumor cell damage through direct destruction, damage to blood vessels, and activation of an immune response.

The foundation of any chemotherapy lies in its selectivity. In PDT, the selectivity arises from increased penetration of the precursor into abnormal cells and perhaps also from decreased metabolism of PpIX into heme in abnormal tissues. The difference in concentration of PpIX between AKs and surrounding normal tissue was shown to be as high as about 10-fold [10], depending on the treatment conditions and precursor used.

Photosensitizers for photodynamic therapy

Two compounds are used for PDT treatment of AKs: 5-ALA (Levulan Kerastick, DUSA Pharmaceuticals, Inc., Wilmington, Massachusetts) and MAL (Metvix, PhotoCure ASA, Oslo, Norway). MAL is believed to be converted into ALA by intracellular esterases.

The intracellular conversion of ALA by the porphyrin pathway results in PpIX, which has significant in vivo absorption bands at approximately 408 nm, 510 nm, 543 nm, 583 nm, and 633 nm [11]. The 408-nm (range, 380–430 nm) "Soret band" is dominant, having up to 15 to 30 fold greater absorption than the longer wavelength "Q-bands" (Fig. 1). The absorption spectrum of PpIX is the most critical, but not the only, determinant in choosing light sources for PDT. The amount of photoactivation depends on how much light reaches the photosensitizer in the tissue. Penetration is affected by the wavelength of the activating light source (longer wavelengths reach deeper into tissues); loss of light due to scatter (especially with shorter wavelengths); and absorption by other chromophores, such as melanin (more significant at shorter wavelengths).

ALA was the original compound developed for use in topical PDT. Usually, it is synthesized in tissues from glycine and succinyl-CoA in the first, rate-limiting step of the porphyrin biosynthetic pathway. By supplying the cells with ready-made ALA, the rate-limiting step is circumvented and porphyrin biosynthesis occurs with accumulation of PpIX. The drawback of ALA is its hydrophilic nature that impedes penetration through the stratum corneum.

MAL is a methyl ester of ALA that was developed to increase its lipophilicity, and, thus, improve penetration though the stratum corneum. Once inside the target cell, MAL undergoes

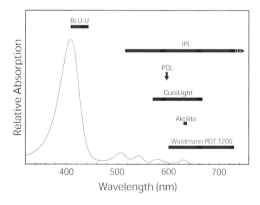

Fig. 1. In vivo absorption spectrum of PpIX and approximate emission wavelengths of common PDT illumination devices.

demethylation to ALA and follows the same sequence of biochemical transformations. Other esters of ALA are in various stages of clinical development [11,12].

Activating light sources in photodynamic therapy for actinic keratoses

As can be inferred from the absorption spectrum of PpIX, there are several options for delivering light in PDT. Although the absorption by the photosensitizer and the depth of penetration are the main determinants, availability of a given light source and other logistics of the application also play a role. The most commonly used photoactivators are blue light sources, intense pulsed light (IPL), pulse-dye laser (PDL), and red light sources. The various trade names of these devices can be a source of confusion because new devices with different spectral characteristics constantly are being developed and marketed. The approximate emission wavelengths also are indicated in Fig. 1.

Blue light corresponds most closely to the "Soret band" of the PpIX absorption spectrum. Two devices, BLU-U (DUSA Pharmaceuticals, Inc.) and ClearLight (Lumenis, Inc., New York, New York) are commercially available. BLU-U consists of parallel fluorescent light tubes that emit most light at about 417 ± 5 nm. ClearLight emits light in the 405- to 420-nm range. Some studies reviewed also used a 400- to 450-nm blue light (Philips, HPM-10, 400 W, Royal Philips Electronics, Amsterdam, the Netherlands).

IPL devices consist of a flash lamp built into an optical treatment head with water-cooled reflective mirrors. IPL is used for multiple applications and is available in many offices [13]. An internal filter removes wavelengths shorter than 500 nm, whereas the water itself often prevents any wavelengths greater than 900 nm from leaving the device. In addition, depending on the device used, various cutoff filters are available that block wavelengths below the given cutoff. Filters are available within the range of 515 to 755 nm. In general, IPL is capable of generating a broad spectrum of light between 515 and 1200 nm. In most cases, IPL will target most of the Q-bands of the PpIX spectrum at the same time.

PDL is a coherent laser light source emitting at 595 nm, and, thus, targets one of the PpIX Q-bands. It seems to be able to deliver the light dose necessary for PDT at subpurpuric doses. The advantage of PDL is that, similarly to IPL, it has numerous other uses, and, therefore, is widely available.

Red light sources are represented by Aktilite and CureLight devices (both by PhotoCure ASA). Aktilite is a light-emitting diode system with peak emission wavelength at 634 ± 3 nm that closely matches the last Q-band of the PpIX absorption spectrum. It is used widely in Europe, and it is the device that is approved by the US Food and Drug Administration (FDA) for use with Metvix PDT. CureLight is a broadband light source covering the spectrum of approximately 570 to 670 nm (centered on 636 nm), which spans two of the longer wavelength Q-bands of the PpIX absorption spectrum.

Waldmann PDT 1200 (Waldmann Medizintechnik, Villingen-Schwenningen, Germany) is a high-pressure metal halide lamp that is reported by the manufacturer to emit light approximately in the 600 to 730 nm range, centered on 630 nm; however, in one study it was reported to be 595 to 700 nm, peaking at 640 nm. The effective target of this system is much like that of CureLight [14].

Other light sources, such as the novel blue light chemiluminescence patches that emit light at 431 to 515 nm [15,16], xenon lamp (615–645 nm), green light (540 ± 15 nm) [17], argon-pumped dye laser (630 nm) [18,19], halogen lamp with a red filter [20], and even a slide projector with or without a filter [4,21], have been used.

Factors determining the dose of photodynamic therapy

Light dose

PDT depends on the production of singlet oxygen and free radicals, and the amounts of those reactive species in and around the lesion determine the outcome of therapy. Assuming adequate levels of molecular oxygen in the tissues, PDT dose is the product of local PpIX concentration and fluence (amount of light, J/cm^2) delivered at wavelengths absorbed by PpIX. It was shown recently, however, that there is a relationship between fluence rate (ie, the rate of light delivery, W/cm^2) and the outcome of PDT, where lower fluence rates over longer times afford better outcomes. This effect most likely is due to oxygen depletion at higher fluence rates, at which the assumption made above would be violated. [22,23] Therefore, PDT dose is most appropriately thought of as the total cytotoxic and immune effect that is determined by the amount of reactive oxygen species created by the complex interplay of molecular oxygen availability, PpIX concentration, total dose of light, and rate of light delivery.

Photosensitizer application and its penetration

For PDT to be effective, the photosensitizer precursors have to penetrate into the target tissue and accumulation of PpIX must occur. Penetration is retarded by stratum corneum, the thickness of which varies among different lesions and in different individuals. Gentle curettage, light chemical peels, microdermabrasion, or pretreatment with acetone all help the precursors to reach deeper into the skin, which increases PDT efficacy. Presence of extensive photodamage, abrasions, or inflammation are expected to afford better percutaneous absorption. The time of application varies between the protocols, from as short as 1 hour to about 14 to 18 hours, although the need for long incubation times has been challenged [24]. MAL is said to penetrate stratum corneum more readily because of its lipophilic nature.

Protoporphyrin IX accumulation

Neoplastic cells accumulate PpIX more readily than do surrounding normal tissues. This has been attributed to increased cellular permeability and slower clearance and metabolism in abnormal cells. The differential absorption seems to be more pronounced during the first few hours after application [10]. It is possible that this selectivity will be enhanced in the future by using further ALA derivatives [25].

Efficacy of photodynamic therapy in treatment of actinic keratoses

The efficacy of ALA and MAL-PDT has been demonstrated in numerous clinical trials. Several recent, large trials are summarized in Table 1 to exemplify the range of response rates.

As part of the phase III clinical trials in 1997, DUSA Pharmaceuticals, Inc. completed two multicenter studies (total of 243 patients) to assess Levulan Kerastick (ALA) and blue light (BLU-U) at 10 J/cm^2 in the treatment of AKs on the face and scalp. If complete response was not obtained after one session, patients were retreated after 8 weeks. At 12 weeks of follow-up, 72% achieved complete clearance and 88% cleared at least 75% of the lesions [26].

PDT using MAL was compared with cryotherapy in a randomized study in Europe that involved 193 patients who had 699 AKs on the face and scalp. MAL was applied for 3 hours and followed by illumination with red light (570–670 nm) at 75 J/cm^2; the treatment was repeated 1 week later in 8% of cases. Cryotherapy was performed using double freeze-thaw cycles of liquid nitrogen. At 3 months follow-up, complete response was achieved in 69% of lesions compared with 75% for cryosurgery; however, the cosmetic outcome of PDT was superior [27].

In another study that was conducted in Australia, 204 patients who had face and scalp AKs were randomized to cryotherapy, placebo, or two sessions of MAL-PDT treatment with red light (570–670 nm) at 75 J/cm^2, 1 week apart. The outcome was assessed after 3 months. Complete remission rate was superior for PDT (91%) versus cryosurgery (68%) or placebo (30%). Again, the cosmetic outcome was superior with PDT [28].

A multicenter, randomized, double-blind, placebo-controlled study of 80 patients who had facial and scalp AKs was conducted in United States. MAL-PDT was compared with placebo using red light with similar parameters as in trials described above. Complete response rate was observed in 89% of lesions, compared with only 38% with placebo. An excellent cosmetic outcome was reported in 91% of patients, when rated by an investigator. When evaluated by patients, 69% rated their outcome as excellent and 22% rated their outcome as good [29].

ALA-PDT for AK treatment was assessed recently in a large, randomized, investigator-blinded, placebo-controlled study that involved 243 patients who had a total of 1403 AKs on scalp and face. Patients were randomized to receive ALA (Levulan Kerastick) or vehicle, followed 14 to 18 hours later by illumination with blue light (BLU-U) at 5 to 10 J/cm^2, depending on patient tolerance (most received 10 J/cm^2). At 8 weeks, 30% of patients who did not respond completely were retreated. At 12 weeks, complete response rate was observed in 91% of the lesions that were treated with ALA. Seventy-three percent of patients experienced clearing of all of their lesions, whereas a clearance rate of at least 75% was observed in 89% of patients. The major side effect observed was moderate to severe discomfort, but only 3% of patients discontinued the therapy for this reason [30].

The FDA-approved protocol calls for two MAL-PDT treatments that are performed 1

Table 1
Recently published large studies evaluating efficacy of photodynamic therapy in treatment of actinic keratoses

Study	Study design	No. of participants	Photosensitizer and application time	Light source and parameters	No. of treatments	Follow-up	Outcome
Tarstedt et al 2005 [31]	Randomized trial of one vs. two PDT sessions	211	MAL, 3 hr under occlusion	LED light, 634 ± 3 nm, 37 J/cm^2 at 50 mW/cm^2	1 vs. 2	3 mo	CR 81% for single Tx. CR 87% for double Tx.
Piacquadio et al 2004 [30]	Randomized, investigator-blinded, placebo-controlled	243	ALA, 14–18 hr	Blue light (417 ± 5 nm), 5–10 J/cm^2 at 10 mW/cm^2 (minimum 500 s)	1–2	12 wk	CR = 91% lesions
Pariser et al 2003 [29]	Double-blind, randomized, placebo-controlled	80	MAL, 3 hr under occlusion	Red light (570–670 nm), 75 J/cm^2 at 50–200 mW/cm^2	2	3 mo	CR = 89% lesions
Freeman et al 2003 [28]	Randomized, PDT vs. cryotherapy vs. placebo	204	MAL, 3 hr under occlusion	Red light (570–670 nm), 75 J/cm^2 at 50–250 mW/cm^2	2	3 mo	CR = 91% lesions
Szeimies et al 2002 [27]	Randomized, PDT vs. cryotherapy	193	MAL, 3 hr under occlusion	Red light (570–670 nm), 75 J/cm^2 total	1	3 mo	CR = 69% lesions

Abbreviations: CR, complete response; LED, light-emitting diode; Tx, treatment.

week apart, while the European labeling suggests a single treatment session. One of the most recent studies assessed the need for retreatment in MAL-PDT for AKs [31]. Two hundred and eleven patients with 413 thin to moderately thick AKs were randomized to receive a single MAL-PDT treatment or two treatments 1 week apart. After gentle surface debridement, MAL cream was applied for 3 hours under occlusion, followed by illumination with red light (Aktilite) at 37 J/cm^2. At 3 months of follow-up, complete response rate after a single treatment was similar to that observed after double treatment protocol (81% versus 87%). Retreatment of nonresponding lesions in patients who originally received only one session increased the efficacy from 81% to 92%. Further analysis of the data revealed that although the efficacy of a single- or two-treatment schedule (without retreatment) was the same in thin AKs, a significant difference was observed in moderately thick lesions (70% versus 84%). Single-treatment protocol also enjoyed higher patient satisfaction (68% versus 55%).

Treatment of actinic keratoses in transplant recipients

AKs present a special situation in transplant recipients. Forty percent of transplant patients encounter premalignant skin tumors within the first 5 years after transplantation, and the risk increases with the time of immunosuppressive treatment [32]. Because the lesions often are multiple and occur in visible areas, the standard treatment methods that can lead to scarring and poor cosmetic outcomes often are less than optimal. Thus, topical use of PDT has been proposed as a promising therapeutic alternative. Effectiveness of ALA-PDT was assessed in an open prospective study that consisted of 20 patients who had undergone transplant and 20 control immunocompetent subjects who presented with AKs and Bowen's disease. 20% ALA in oil-water emulsion was applied for 5 hours under occlusion, followed by irradiation with visible light (Waldmann PDT 1200) for a total of 75 J/cm^2. In some patients, the PDT session was repeated 1 week later. Overall complete response in patients who had undergone transplants was 86% at 4 weeks (versus 94% in controls), but it decreased to 48% at 48 weeks (versus 72% in controls) [33]. The same group assessed MAL-PDT in a prospective, randomized, double-blind, placebo-controlled study that consisted of 17 transplant recipients with a total of

129 AKs. Two lesional areas were identified in each patient and randomized to receive two consecutive treatments of topical PDT 1 week apart, using MAL or placebo cream. After curettage of crusts and scale, MAL cream was applied to the lesions under occlusion for 3 hours. This was followed by irradiation with visible light (Waldmann PDT 1200) for a total of 75 J/cm^2. At 16 weeks of follow up, complete response was seen in 76% of areas that were treated actively, and a partial or complete response was seen in 94% of areas. No response was noted with placebo [34].

Based on these studies and other similar observations, PDT has emerged as a promising modality to prevent progression of AKs to SCC, which is the most common posttransplantation malignancy in white populations [35]. This promise, however, has been overshadowed by a recent trial that focused specifically on the preventive effect of PDT on the development of new SCCs in transplant recipients. In this randomized, controlled study, 40 transplant patients received ALA-PDT to one randomly assigned hand and forearm, but not to the other. ALA was applied as a topical cream to the whole treatment field under occlusion for 4 hours, without previous removal of the scale. Illumination was attained with a 400- to 450-nm light source (Philips HPM-10, 400 W) for a total dose of 5.5 to 6 J/cm^2. The treatment was repeated 6 months later in half of the patients. During the 2-year follow-up period, there was no statistically significant difference between areas that were and were not treated with PDT, in terms of the number of SCCs (a total of 25 lesions was observed) [36]. Although treatment protocol may not have been optimal in this study, it is becoming clear that PDT does not enjoy the same excellent efficacy in transplant recipients that is observed in immunocompetent patients. One of the reasons for poorer outcomes is that success of PDT, in addition to direct killing and vascular damage, likely relies on induction of innate and adaptive immune responses [37].

Further benefits of photodynamic therapy over other treatments for actinic keratoses

Treatment of premalignant lesions and prevention of progression to SCC is the main objective of the PDT treatments described. It was shown, however, that PDT—performed with IPL as the source of illumination—also has improved appearance of telangiectasias, pigmentary irregularities,

---

Box 1. Outline of aminolevulinic acid photodynamic therapy for actinic keratoses

The surface of the AK is scrubbed with acetone or debrided gently by curettage, EKG tape, or microdermabrasion [9].

For ALA-PDT using Levulan Kerastick, the stick is crushed and mixed for at least 3 minutes to allow dissolution of ALA, in accordance with the manufacturer's insert [26].

The preparation is applied directly to the target lesions by dabbing the skin with the wet applicator tip of the Kerastick. Approximately 5 mm of perilesional skin is included, but the technique also can be used for large field treatment.

Patients should not expose themselves to sun or intense light after the application.

Sufficient time is allowed for incubation. The product monograph suggests 14 to 18 hours but shorter incubation times of 1 to 2 hours have been shown to be effective and more practical.

For pain control, nonsteroidal anti-inflammatory drugs or acetaminophen can be used, in conjunction with ice packs and air cooling. Topical anesthetics do not seem to provide much benefit [39].

Before illumination, the area is cleaned with water or normal saline and patted dry. Woods light may be used to confirm PpIX fluorescence in the targeted lesions, but this may not be obvious at shorter incubation times.

Illumination is achieved with the light source of choice. The Levulan Kerastick product monograph suggests activation with BLU-U light source at 10 J/cm^2 for 16 minutes, 40 seconds. The patient and the personnel should wear appropriate protective eyewear.

Patients should avoid sun and intense light for 24 to 48 hours following illumination. Physical sunscreens can be used as a supplementary measure. Noncompliance may lead to severe phototoxic reactions.

Lesions that have not resolved in 8 weeks may be retreated. Regular follow-up is recommended.

Box 2. Outline of methyl aminolevulinate photodynamic therapy for actinic keratoses

The surface of the AK is debrided gently by curettage to remove hyperkeratotic scales and crusts.

A 1-mm layer of MAL cream (Metvix) is applied directly to the target lesions and 5- to 10-mm perilesional area with a spatula. The area is covered with an occlusive dressing, such as Tegaderm (3M, St. Paul, Minnesota), and incubated for 3 hours.

Patients should avoid sun or intense light after the application, although the cream provides a certain amount of shielding during incubation time.

After 3 hours, the dressing is removed and the area is cleaned with saline. Illumination is achieved with the light source of choice. With Aktilite, a total dose of 37 J/cm^2 is used over about 9 minutes. The distance between the light source and the skin surface is kept at about 5 to 8 cm. The patient and the personnel should wear appropriate protective eyewear.

For pain control, nonsteroidal anti-inflammatory drugs or acetaminophen can be used, in conjunction with ice packs and air cooling. Topical anesthetics do not seem to provide any benefit [39].

Following illumination, patients should protect themselves from sun and intense light for at least 48 hours. Physical sun blocks can be used but are no substitution for the patient's compliance.

According to the FDA-approved protocol, the treatment with MAL should be repeated in 7 days.

and coarseness of skin texture [38]. Such added benefits may improve patient compliance and satisfaction.

Practical strategies for using photodynamic therapy in treatment of actinic keratoses

The procedure of performing PDT for AKs varies, depending on the patient, photosensitizer precursor, and the particular light source used (Boxes 1 and 2). Before the procedure, biopsy or excision should be performed on any suspected SCCs, basal cell carcinomas, or melanomas, because superficial treatment of those lesions may lead to deep recurrence. The risks, benefits, and alternative treatments must be discussed with the patient. A certain level of phototoxicity is desired, and patients should be warned to expect some degree of erythema, burning sensation, vesiculation, crusting, and erosions. Severe phototoxic reactions may need rescue treatment.

Summary

ALA-PDT is an extremely useful addition to our traditional armamentarium of AK treatments. It offers versatility and superior cosmetic outcomes, while delivering excellent clinical results. Two topical photosensitizer precursors, 5-ALA and MAL, are available commercially. Specialized equipment is commercially available (eg, BLU-U), but illumination also can be achieved with various other light sources, including PDL and IPL, which circumvents the need for specialized equipment. The technique can be used for spot as well as field treatment, offering to treat clinically elusive early lesions successfully.

Acknowledgments

We would like to acknowledge the help of Anna Kalisiak, graphic designer, in the preparation of this manuscript.

References

[1] Gupta AK, Cooper EA, Feldman SR, et al. A survey of office visits for actinic keratosis as reported by NAMCS, 1990–1999. National Ambulatory Medical Care Survey. Cutis 2002;70(2 Suppl):8–13.

[2] Lebwohl M. Actinic keratosis: epidemiology and progression to squamous cell carcinoma. Br J Dermatol 2003;149(Suppl 66):31–3.

[3] Glogau RG. The risk of progression to invasive disease. J Am Acad Dermatol 2000;42(1 Pt 2):23–4.

[4] Kennedy JC, Pottier RH, Pross DC. Photodynamic therapy with endogenous protoporphyrin IX: basic principles and present clinical experience. J Photochem Photobiol B 1990;6(1–2):143–8.

[5] Gold MH, Nestor MS. Current treatments of actinic keratosis. J Drugs Dermatol 2006;5(2 Suppl):17–25.

[6] Cockerell CJ, Wharton JR. New histopathological classification of actinic keratosis (incipient intraepidermal squamous cell carcinoma). J Drugs Dermatol 2005;4(4):462–7.

[7] Davis DA, Donahue JP, Bost JE, et al. The diagnostic concordance of actinic keratosis and squamous cell carcinoma. J Cutan Pathol 2005;32(8):546–51.

[8] Gold MH. The evolving role of aminolevulinic acid hydrochloride with photodynamic therapy in photoaging. Cutis 2002;69(6 Suppl):8–13.

[9] Goldman MP. Photodynamic therapy. Philadelphia: Elsevier; 2005.

[10] Angell-Petersen E, Sorensen R, Warloe T, et al. Porphyrin formation in actinic keratosis and basal cell carcinoma after topical application of methyl 5-aminolevulinate. J Invest Dermatol 2006;126(2):265–71.

[11] Juzenas P, Juzeniene A, Kaalhus O, et al. Noninvasive fluorescence excitation spectroscopy during application of 5-aminolevulinic acid in vivo. Photochem Photobiol Sci 2002;1(10):745–8.

[12] Fotinos N, Campo MA, Popowycz F, et al. 5-Aminolevulinic acid aerivatives in photomedicine: basics, application and perspectives. Photochem Photobiol 2006;82(4):994–1015.

[13] Goldman MP, Weiss RA, Weiss MA. Intense pulsed light as a nonablative approach to photoaging. Dermatol Surg 2005;31(9 Pt 2):1179–87.

[14] Varma S, Wilson H, Kurwa HA, et al. Bowen's disease, solar keratoses and superficial basal cell carcinomas treated by photodynamic therapy using a large-field incoherent light source. Br J Dermatol 2001;144(3):567–74.

[15] Zelickson B, Counters J, Coles C, et al. Light patch: preliminary report of a novel form of blue light delivery for the treatment of actinic keratosis. Dermatol Surg 2005;31(3):375–8.

[16] Wolf P, Rieger E, Kerl H. Topical photodynamic therapy with endogenous porphyrins after application of 5-aminolevulinic acid. An alternative treatment modality for solar keratoses, superficial squamous cell carcinomas, and basal cell carcinomas? J Am Acad Dermatol 1993;28(1):17–21.

[17] Morton CA, Whitehurst C, Moore JV, et al. Comparison of red and green light in the treatment of Bowen's disease by photodynamic therapy. Br J Dermatol 2000;143(4):767–72.

[18] Calzavara-Pinton PG. Repetitive photodynamic therapy with topical delta-aminolaevulinic acid as an appropriate approach to the routine treatment of superficial non-melanoma skin tumours. J Photochem Photobiol B 1995;29(1):53–7.

[19] Jeffes EW, McCullough JL, Weinstein GD, et al. Photodynamic therapy of actinic keratosis with topical 5-aminolevulinic acid. A pilot dose-ranging study. Arch Dermatol 1997;133(6):727–32.

[20] Fijan S, Honigsmann H, Ortel B. Photodynamic therapy of epithelial skin tumours using delta-aminolaevulinic acid and desferrioxamine. Br J Dermatol 1995;133(2):282–8.

[21] Fink-Puches R, Hofer A, Smolle J, et al. Primary clinical response and long-term follow-up of solar keratoses treated with topically applied 5-aminolevulinic acid and irradiation by different wave bands of light. J Photochem Photobiol B 1997;41(1–2): 145–51.

[22] Ericson MB, Sandberg C, Stenquist B, et al. Photodynamic therapy of actinic keratosis at varying fluence rates: assessment of photobleaching, pain and primary clinical outcome. Br J Dermatol 2004; 151(6):1204–12.

[23] Henderson BW, Busch TM, Snyder JW. Fluence rate as a modulator of PDT mechanisms. Lasers Surg Med 2006;38(5):489–93.

[24] Touma D, Yaar M, Whitehead S, et al. A trial of short incubation, broad-area photodynamic therapy for facial actinic keratoses and diffuse photodamage. Arch Dermatol 2004;140(1):33–40.

[25] Perotti C, Fukuda H, DiVenosa G, et al. Porphyrin synthesis from ALA derivatives for photodynamic therapy. In vitro and in vivo studies. Br J Cancer 2004;90(8):1660–5.

[26] DUSA Pharmaceuticals. Levulan Kerastick (aminolevulinic acid HCl) for topical solution, 20%. Product Insert. 2004.

[27] Szeimies RM, Karrer S, Radakovic-Fijan S, et al. Photodynamic therapy using topical methyl 5-aminolevulinate compared with cryotherapy for actinic keratosis: a prospective, randomized study. J Am Acad Dermatol 2002;47(2):258–62.

[28] Freeman M, Vinciullo C, Francis D, et al. A comparison of photodynamic therapy using topical methyl aminolevulinate (Metvix) with single cycle cryotherapy in patients with actinic keratosis: a prospective, randomized study. J Dermatolog Treat 2003;14(2):99–106.

[29] Pariser DM, Lowe NJ, Stewart DM, et al. Photodynamic therapy with topical methyl aminolevulinate for actinic keratosis: results of a prospective randomized multicenter trial. J Am Acad Dermatol 2003;48(2):227–32.

[30] Piacquadio DJ, Chen DM, Farber HF, et al. Photodynamic therapy with aminolevulinic acid topical solution and visible blue light in the treatment of multiple actinic keratoses of the face and scalp: investigator-blinded, phase 3, multicenter trials. Arch Dermatol 2004;140(1):41–6.

[31] Tarstedt M, Rosdahl I, Berne B, et al. A randomized multicenter study to compare two treatment regimens of topical methyl aminolevulinate (Metvix)-PDT in actinic keratosis of the face and scalp. Acta Derma Venereol 2005;85(5):424–8.

[32] Stockfleth E, Ulrich C, Meyer T, et al. Epithelial malignancies in organ transplant patients: clinical presentation and new methods of treatment. Recent Results Cancer Res 2002;160:251–8.

[33] Dragieva G, Hafner J, Dummer R, et al. Topical photodynamic therapy in the treatment of actinic keratoses and Bowen's disease in transplant recipients. Transplantation 2004;77(1):115–21.

[34] Dragieva G, Prinz BM, Hafner J, et al. A randomized controlled clinical trial of topical photodynamic therapy with methyl aminolaevulinate in the treatment of actinic keratoses in transplant recipients. Br J Dermatol 2004;151(1):196–200.

[35] Sheil AG, Disney AP, Mathew TH, et al. De novo malignancy emerges as a major cause of morbidity and late failure in renal transplantation. Transplant Proc 1993;25(1 Pt 2):1383–4.

[36] de Graaf YG, Kennedy C, Wolterbeek R, et al. Photodynamic therapy does not prevent cutaneous squamous-cell carcinoma in organ-transplant recipients: results of a randomized-controlled trial. J Invest Dermatol 2006;126(3):569–74.

[37] Oseroff A. PDT as a cytotoxic agent and biological response modifier: Implications for cancer prevention and treatment in immunosuppressed and immunocompetent patients. J Invest Dermatol 2006; 126(3):542–4.

[38] Avram DK, Goldman MP. Effectiveness and safety of ALA-IPL in treating actinic keratoses and photodamage. J Drugs Dermatol 2004;3(1 Suppl): S36–9.

[39] Langan SM, Collins P. Randomized, double-blind, placebo-controlled prospective study of the efficacy of topical anaesthesia with a eutetic mixture of lignocaine 2.5% and prilocaine 2.5% for topical 5-aminolaevulinic acid-photodynamic therapy for extensive scalp actinic keratoses. Br J Dermatol 2006;154(1): 146–9.

ELSEVIER
SAUNDERS

DERMATOLOGIC
CLINICS

Dermatol Clin 25 (2007) 25–33

Aminolevulinic Acid Photodynamic Therapy for Actinic Keratoses/Actinic Cheilitis/Acne: Vascular Lasers

Macrene Alexiades-Armenakas, MD, PhD*

Yale University School of Medicine, New Haven, CT, USA

Since its inception more than a century ago, modern photodynamic therapy (PDT) has been conducted using a variety of photosensitizers and light sources. Initially, systemic photosensitizers, such as hematoporphyrin [1], were combined with broadband light sources in the red and blue range of the spectrum to treat a variety of cutaneous neoplasms [2,3]. Until 1995, when porfirin sodium was approved by the US Food and Drug Administration (FDA) for treatment of esophageal carcinoma, the treatment was experimental and was associated with marked side effects (eg, prolonged photosensitivity). The introduction of topical 5-aminolevulinic acid (ALA) for cutaneous disorders in the 1980s eliminated the problem of generalized cutaneous photosensitivity [4,5]. Topical ALA was used in combination with red and blue light, the latter of which achieved FDA clearance for treating actinic keratoses (AK) in 1997. With the advent of lasers over the past 2 decades, red and, less often, blue light lasers have been used with topical ALA to treat cutaneous neoplasms and inflammatory disorders (eg, acne vulgaris); however, these previous light sources were associated with significant side effects (eg, discomfort, crusting, blistering, erythema, dyspigmentation, localized phototoxic reactions) [6]. The combination of newer laser and light sources, the long-pulsed pulsed dye laser (LP PDL) and intense pulsed light (IPL), with topical ALA PDT has achieved enhanced efficacy and rapid treatment and recovery, while diminishing unwanted side effects [7]. In particular, LP PDL PDT has been shown to be safe and effective in the treatment of AK, actinic cheilitis (AC), photodamage, and acne vulgaris, with minimal discomfort, rapid treatment and recovery, and excellent posttreatment cosmesis [6].

Background of earlier light sources

The light source used for PDT is determined by the absorption spectrum of the photosensitizer, and the wavelength and penetration depth of the light. The porphyrins, which are the foremost class of photosensitizers in PDT, absorb light maximally in the Soret band ranging from 360 nm to 400 nm, with additional smaller peaks, the Q bands, between 500 nm and 635 nm [8,9]. 5-ALA is converted within target cells into the photosensitizer protoporphyrin IX (PpIX), which has an absorption spectrum with a large blue peak at 417 nm and a small red peak at 650 nm [10]. The depth of penetration increases directly proportionally to wavelength across the visible spectrum; 50% penetration is 80 μm for a 355-nm laser and increases to 1200 μm for a 694-nm laser [11]. Noncoherent light sources, while expected to achieve less optical penetration because of scatter, have been reported to achieve good penetration—up to 5 mm for 630-nm light and 1 to 2 cm for 700-nm to 800-nm light [12–14]. Because of these two factors, most research has focused on light sources that emit wavelengths in the blue range, which is absorbed optimally by porphyrins, and the red range, which is absorbed less well, but has a deeper penetration depth [9].

Broad-spectrum light sources: blue and red light

The light sources that were used initially in PDT predominantly were broad-spectrum light

* 880 Fifth Avenue, New York, NY 11021.
E-mail address: dralexiades@nyderm.org.

0733-8635/07/$ - see front matter © 2006 Elsevier Inc. All rights reserved.
doi:10.1016/j.det.2006.09.003

sources in combination with systemic photosensitizers. In the 1940s, a quartz lamp was used in combination with hematoporphyrin to treat tumors [2]. In the 1960s, a xenon arc lamp (600–660 nm) was combined with hematoporphyrin derivative [15,16]. In the 1970s and 1980s, xenon arc lamps, slide projectors emitting 400 nm to 650 nm using red filters, and halogen lamps emitting 600 nm to 800 nm were combined with hematoporphyrin derivative to treat skin neoplasms [17–19]. In the 1990s, research with noncoherent light sources in the red and blue range for PDT continued [20–22]. Since 1990, when topical ALA was introduced in combination with a tungsten slide projector with a red 600-nm cut-off filter for the treatment of cutaneous neoplasms and AK, topical ALA became the predominant photosensitizer for cutaneous use [5]. The light sources that were used initially were in the red range, such as tungsten light sources with red filters [5,23,24], xenon arc lamps (600–720 nm) [25], or halogen lamps (570-690 nm) [26]. Finally, in the late 1990s, blue light became the predominant light source studied with topical ALA for the treatment of AK because of their superficial location in the skin; more recently, it has been applied to the treatment of photodamage and acne vulgaris [27–30]. This method achieved FDA approval for the treatment of AK in 1997 [27]. Methylated ALA has been studied almost exclusively with red light for the treatment of basal cell carcinoma and AK [31–35]. The aforementioned light sources have been associated with significant side effects, such as pain, discomfort, blistering, and crusting. Thus, noncoherent broad-spectrum light sources in the red and blue wavelengths, in conjunction with systemic or topical porphyrins, were the earliest and most frequently used light sources in PDT for cutaneous diseases, although they are associated with significant side effects.

Red and blue lasers in photodynamic therapy

Lasers were introduced and reported extensively for use with PDT in the 1990s. They were predominantly of red, and to a lesser extent blue, wavelengths, and were used for internal and cutaneous conditions. Lasers provided several advantages, including the ability to be coupled to fiber optics for access to internal tumors; the ability to select a specific wavelength and maximize penetration depth; and the ability to achieve higher irradiances, which decreased exposure times [36]. Most lasers that are used for PDT with systemic photosensitizers have been in the red range, including tunable dye (630 nm), gold vapor (628 nm), and red diode (688 nm) [37]. Less frequently, lasers in the blue range, such as argon (488 nm and 514 nm), were used [38]. Topical PDT also has been combined mainly with red lasers, such as the copper vapor-dye (630 nm), the neodymium: yttrium aluminum garnet (Nd:YAG) laser (630 nm), the argon ion–dye laser (630 nm) [39–44], and an argon pumped-dye laser (633 nm) [45].

Red lasers and light, although effective, have been associated with significant side effects when used with PDT. Blistering, erythema, edema, and dyspigmentation were reported in multiple studies of broadband red light (550–700 nm) and red diode (635 nm) laser-mediated PDT for acne vulgaris [46,47]. Additional studies of red light (660 nm), red laser at 635 nm, and red light at 600 nm to 700 nm reproduced these findings, noting significant pain and discomfort during treatment in addition to postoperative blistering, crusting, and dyspigmentation [48–51]. Thus, red lasers and light in combination with ALA PDT have been effective in treating cutaneous neoplasms and acne vulgaris, but with significant side effects.

Optimizing the light source for cutaneous photodynamic therapy

The ideal light source in cutaneous PDT should (1) be absorbed well by the photosensitizer, (2) achieve a desirable penetration depth, thereby reaching its target, (3) have an adequate fluence and duration to drive the PDT reaction, (4) be rapid to administer, and (5) have minimal discomfort, be purpura-free, with minimal erythema, rapid recovery, and no risk for crusting or dyspigmentation. The aforementioned light and laser sources achieved some, but not all, of these objectives, often with significant side effects. One plausible explanation is that the side effects of discomfort during the lengthy illumination process, and of prolonged posttreatment erythema, crusting, and dyspigmentation are dependent upon the light source. Therefore, an optimal light source would be one of adequate light energy in less time, and with greater selectivity for the target condition and minimal background photosensitivity in surrounding normal skin.

Long-pulsed pulsed dye laser–mediated photodynamic therapy

In the course of addressing this hypothesis, the absorption spectrum of PpIX was analyzed;

a peak at 575 nm was noted among the Q bands [10]. In a previous study, the PDL at 585 nm was used in conjunction with topical 20% ALA PDT for the treatment of AK with clearance rates of 79% at 1 month follow-up, but with cosmetically unacceptable purpura [52]. Subsequently, it was noted that 595 nm is present on the side of this Q band, and the LP PDL (595 nm) was selected as an alternate light source for ALA PDT [7]. The LP PDL uniquely meets the criteria of an ideal PDT light source. It has the advantages of variable pulse duration in the nonpurpuric range; a longer wavelength with greater penetration depth as compared with blue light; dynamic cooling spray to minimize discomfort; large 10-mm spot size, and great rapidity of treatment with a firing speed of 1 Hz. Thus, the LP PDL was investigated in an attempt to improve patient acceptance of ALA PDT.

Actinic keratoses

In the first study of LP PDL PDT of 41 patients who had AK, ALA was applied for 3 hours versus 14 to 18 hours [7]. This was followed by LP PDL irradiation at 595 nm, 7.5 J/cm^2 fluence, 10-millisecond pulse duration, 10-mm spot size, and dynamic cooling spray of 30 milliseconds with 30-millisecond delay. The mean percent head AK lesions cleared was approximately 90% at 8 months of follow-up, which was comparable to other treatment modalities, such as topical fluorouracil or PDT with blue light [27]. In addition to high efficacy rates, LP PDL–mediated PDT achieved rapid treatment times of less than 5 minutes for full head; minimal discomfort; and minimal posttreatment erythema, which resolved within 5 days. There was no incidence of blistering, crusting, or dyspigmentation. Of import, this was the first clinical study to demonstrate that short-incubation (3 hours) ALA was as effective as long-incubation (14–18 hours) ALA [7]. These findings have been reproduced with short-incubation ALA and blue light [29]. An example of a patient who had numerous AK before, immediately following, and 2 weeks after one treatment with LP PDL PDT is shown in Fig. 1.

Photodamage

An evident extension of this application for AK is the use of LP PDL PDT for the closely related condition of photodamage. Because photodamage or actinic damage lies on a continuum

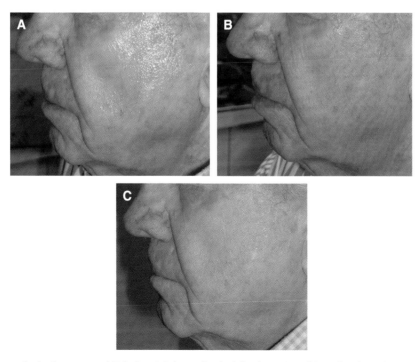

Fig. 1. Patient who had numerous AK before (*A*), immediately following (*B*), and 2 weeks after (*C*) one treatment with LP PDL PDT.

with AK, this result was not surprising. Although improvement in texture and erythema were expected from AK clearance, improvements in fine rhytides and lentigines also were observed. Photographs of a patient who had extensive photodamage before, immediately following LP PDL-mediated PDT, and after 2 weeks are shown in Fig. 1. Treatment of photoaging with LP PDL PDT has been reported [53]. Further research in this area of PDT mainly has used the IPL in conjunction with topical ALA PDT, given the well-documented efficacy of IPL alone for this application. The addition of ALA has been used to accelerate photorejuvenation and decrease treatment numbers [54,55].

Actinic cheilitis

ALA PDT activated by LP PDL (595 nm) subsequently was found to be safe and effective with minimal side effects for a related precancerous condition, AC, for which alternative treatment options have been of limited efficacy [56]. In a study of 21 patients who had refractory AC, 20% topical ALA was applied for a short 2-hour incubation, followed by two passes of LP PDL (595 nm) at 7 to 7.5 J/cm^2 fluence, 10-millisecond pulse duration, 10-mm spot size, and dynamic cooling spray of 30 milliseconds with 30-millisecond delay [56]. Complete clearance was achieved in 13 of 19 (68%) patients following a mean of 1.8 treatments. Among those, 7 of 13 cleared after one treatment, 2 of 13 cleared after two treatments, and 1 of 13 cleared after three treatments, with a mean follow-up of 4.1 months (range, 1–12). Side effects were minimal with none-to-mild pain, slight-to-moderate erythema that lasted less than 3 days, and no crusting, purpura, or scarring. Treatment time was extremely rapid (<1 minute) [56]. LP PDL PDT for the treatment of AC achieved the advantages of rapid incubation, treatment, and recovery times; minimal discomfort; excellent cosmetic outcome; and good efficacy rates, although multiple treatments may be required for complete clearing. An example of a patient who had biopsy-proven AC, with complete resolution following a single treatment with LP PDL-mediated PDT, is shown in Fig. 2.

Mechanism of long-pulsed pulsed dye laser–mediated photodynamic therapy of actinic diseases

Classically, the PDT reaction has involved marked erythema and crusting, and this response

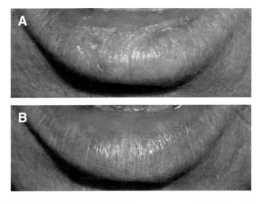

Fig. 2. Patient who had biopsy-proven AC (*A*), with complete resolution of AC following a single treatment with LP PDL–mediated PDT (*B*).

was considered to be an integral component of its effectiveness. At the same time, however, this reaction made PDT tolerated less well by patients. The rapid recovery and minimal erythema that are observed following LP PDL–mediated ALA PDT of AK, AC, and photodamage suggest a unique mechanism of tumor clearance that is more selective to the target cells and less dependent upon an inflammatory response or nonspecific skin necrosis [6]. One potential explanation for this finding is that LP PDL elicits a novel PDT response, perhaps triggering apoptosis that is devoid of any significant accompanying inflammatory response or ischemic necrosis.

To understand the classic "PDT reaction" and the cause of the crusting that is observed, one must recall the early discovery by Von Tappeiner (1903) that PDT is an oxygen-dependent process [57,58]. PDT is mediated by oxygen-dependent photochemical reactions, during which photosensitizers are excited from the ground state to a higher-energy singlet state, and, finally, a reactive triplet state [59]. From the triplet state, the photosensitizer reacts with oxygen to form a reactive species (eg, singlet oxygen [the type II reaction]) or directly with a cellular target to form free radicals or radical ions (type I reaction). Once singlet oxygen or free radicals have been generated, their principal targets seem to be the cellular and mitochondrial membranes, and endoplasmic reticulum, which leads to cell death. The mechanism of cell death in this specific PDT reaction seems to be by apoptosis; it has been demonstrated in cell culture experiments of carcinoma cell lines following PDT with ALA and other photosensitizers [59]. Ischemic necrosis from vascular compromise and local tissue hypoxia has been implicated as a main culprit in the degree of PDT reaction [59]. Therefore, the selectivity of the treatment may depend upon the localization of photosensitizer in target cells, and the degree of ischemia generated.

Strategies that may improve PDT effects by allowing adequate tissue oxygenation include using lower irradiances, which decrease the rate of oxygen consumption, or dividing light exposure into a series of shorter exposures to allow for tissue reoxygenation. The latter strategy is used by lasers, although LP PDL seems to clear target efficiently with less inflammation and no necrosis as compared with red lasers. A potential explanation for the efficient clearance of precancerous cells without the degree of tissue damage that is observed with other light sources may be that LP PDL triggers apoptosis, and the 10-millisecond light pulses that are delivered at 1 Hz allow for adequate reoxygenation between pulses, such that ischemic necrosis is averted. Further investigation is warranted to test this hypothesis. In summary, LP PDL PDT may achieve target cell clearance through apoptosis while minimizing side effects by averting the inflammatory response and tissue ischemia, a plausible theory that deserves further research.

Acne vulgaris

Initially, the rationale for PDT to treat acne vulgaris was based upon the fact that porphyrins are produced in small quantities by *Propionibacterium acnes* [60]. In obstructed follicles, the anaerobic bacterium proliferates and incites inflammation. When exposed to light, a PDT reaction occurs in the acne vulgaris lesions, which causes singlet oxygen production and bacterial destruction [61]. Blue light without ALA has been of modest efficacy in the treatment of acne vulgaris, presumably because of its poor depth of skin penetration [48]. In contrast, red light—although less effective at porphyrin photoactivation—penetrates deeper, and when combined with blue light, increases effectiveness [48].

In addition, it was observed that exogenous ALA concentrates in sebaceous units; therefore, topical ALA was added to increase the efficacy of PDT for acne vulgaris. When ALA was injected intraperitoneally into mice, PpIX accumulated in the sebaceous glands of normal skin, and light of the appropriate wavelength destroyed sebaceous glands [62]. Topical application of ALA induced selective PpIX fluorescence in acne vulgaris

lesions with minimal background in surrounding normal skin [46]. PDT with red light was shown to shrink sebaceous glands [46]; however, red light and lasers were among the first light sources used for the treatment of acne vulgaris with PDT and bore significant side effects (eg, blistering, erythema, edema, dyspigmentation) [46–50].

Because LP PDL with ALA PDT was effective in reducing sebaceous hyperplasia [63,64], it was evaluated as an alternative light source for PDT of acne vulgaris. In an initial pilot study, a 50% to 60% reduction in mean acne vulgaris counts was observed after a single treatment, with minimal erythema that lasted for approximately 2 days [63]. Recently, a controlled trial that assessed LP PDL–mediated ALA PDT combined with topical therapy for the treatment of acne vulgaris was completed [65]. The patients in the study were recalcitrant to conventional therapies, including oral isotretinoin, and suffered from acne vulgaris of all types and levels of severity. Short-incubation (45 minutes) ALA followed by LP PDL was compared with blue light, LP PDL alone, and conventional treatment controls. Complete clearance was achieved in all 14 patients who were treated with LP PDL PDT following a mean of three treatments (range, 1–6), and it was maintained at a mean of 6 months (range, 1–13) of follow-up. The mean percent clearance rates per treatment were 77% for LP PDL PDT, 32% for LP PDL alone, and 20% for conventional therapy, which included oral antibiotics and oral contraceptives; all patients were maintained on topical therapy. The blue light arm of the study was curtailed because of recrudescence. Following LP PDL PDT, minimal erythema was observed that lasted for 1 to 2 days, with no incidence of crusting, purpura, scarring, or dyspigmentation [65]. Fig. 3 shows a patient who had acne vulgaris before and following a single treatment with LP PDL PDT. Adequate efficacy with minimal side effects was achieved with LP PDL in combination with ALA PDT and topical therapy; however, a randomized, double-blind, vehicle-controlled trial of monotherapy is pending.

The effectiveness of LP PDL–mediated PDT in treating acne vulgaris seems to be due to the LP PDL energy as well as the ALA PDT component; this may explain its higher efficacy as compared with blue light. The LP PDL alone control in the aforementioned study [63] showed a lesional clearance rate that was superior to the topical medications/oral antibiotics/oral contraceptives control. This supports previous studies that demonstrated

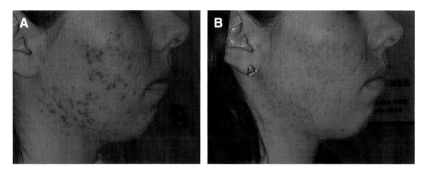

Fig. 3. Patient who had acne vulgaris before (*A*) and following (*B*) a single treatment with LP PDL PDT.

that PDL may be an effective treatment in acne vulgaris [66]. A recent report that suggested that PDL may be ineffective used low fluences of 3 J/cm^2 [67]. In the author's experience—and as shown by the control group in the current study—the fluence that is necessary to achieve efficacy using LP PDL may be higher (ie, 7–7.5 J/cm^2). The mechanisms may involve blood vessel targeting, as well as photothermal effects on sebaceous follicles and weak, but adequate, photoactivation of endogenous porphyrins that are produced by *P acnes* in the sebaceous follicle. Supportive evidence that PDT targets the sebaceous gland is demonstrated well by decreased sebaceous gland size and vacuolization of sebocytes following PDT [46]. Thus, the mechanism of PDT in the treatment of acne vulgaris likely involves direct thermal or photodynamic injury to the sebaceous glands, destruction of *P acnes*, or a facilitation of keratinocyte turnover in the infundibulum [46]. The number of treatments that is needed to achieve acne vulgaris clearance may be due to hormonal factors and the size and activity of the sebaceous glands at baseline, such that multiple sessions are required to achieve adequate destruction of sebaceous gland function.

Lichen sclerosus

PDT has been used to treat inflammatory conditions, and it is effective in the treatment of lichen sclerosus [68,69]. This autoimmune sclerosing disease is characterized by dilated blood vessels in the upper dermis, thinning of the epidermis, and an inflammatory cell infiltrate, which may be due to autoantibody to the extracellular matrix protein ECM-1. Vulvar lichen sclerosus has been treated effectively with topical ALA and blue light [68]. More recently, extragenital lichen sclerosus was cleared completely following three treatments with LP PDL–mediated ALA PDT [69]. The areas treated have remained clear for 2 years (Fig. 4) [67].

Other applications

PDL-mediated PDT has been used to target other cutaneous disorders with a vascular component. It has been investigated for the treatment of

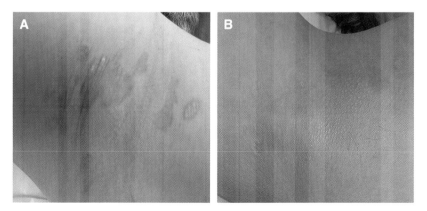

Fig. 4. Patient who had lesions before (*A*) and following (*B*) three treatments, with 2 years' follow-up.

port wine stains [70]. A combined photodynamic and photothermal effect from PDL PDT has been shown to enhance blood vessel injury in vivo [71]. In addition, PDL-mediated PDT has been used to treat verrucae [72].

Summary

Optimizing the light source for PDT has been an integral component to maximizing efficacy and minimizing side effects, and has succeeded in bringing this useful therapeutic modality into the mainstream. Since the beginning of the twentieth century, PDT has evolved from a systemic treatment, with multiple side effects, to its adaptation for cutaneous use as a topical treatment, with minimal side effects for a variety of skin conditions. Although earlier light sources, such as broadband light and lasers in the red and blue range, were effective, they were associated with unwanted side effects. The introduction of newer light sources, such as LP PDL for ALA PDT, has maintained efficacy with an excellent side effect profile. LP PDL PDT is safe and effective in the treatment of AK, AC, photodamage, acne vulgaris, and other dermatologic conditions.

References

[1] Meyer-Betz F. [Investigation of biological (photodynamic) actions of hematoporphyrins and other derivatives of blood and bilirubin]. Dtsch Arch Klin Med 1913;112:476 [in German].

[2] Auler H, Banzer G. Untersucheungen uber die rolle der porphyrine bei geschwulstkranken menschen und tieren. Z Krebsforsch 1942;53:65.

[3] Figge FHJ, Wiland GS, Manganiello LOJ. Cancer detection and therapy: affinity of neoplastic, embryonic and traumatized tissues for porphyrins and metalloporphyrins. Proc Soc Exp Biol Med 1948; 68:640–1.

[4] Malik Z, Lugaci H. Destruction of erythroleukaemic cells by photoactivation of endogenous porphyrins. Br J Cancer 1987;56:589–95.

[5] Kennedy JC, Pottier RH, Pross DC. Photodynamic therapy with endogenous protoporphyrin IX: basic principles and present clinical experience. J Photochem Photobiol B 1990;14:275–92.

[6] Alexiades-Armenakas MR. Laser-mediated photodynamic therapy. Clin Dermatol 2006;24(1):16–25.

[7] Alexiades-Armenakas MR, Geronemus G. Laser-mediated photodynamic therapy of actinic keratoses. Arch Dermatol 2003;139(10):1313–20.

[8] Soret JL. Recherches sur l'absorption des rayons ultra violets par diverses substances [Research on the absorption of ultraviolet rays by diverse substances]. Arch Sci Phys Nat 1883;10:430–85 [in French].

[9] Kurwa HA, Barlow RJ. The role of photodynamic therapy in dermatology. Clin Exp Dermatol 1999; 24(3):143–8.

[10] Pottier RH, Chow YFA, LaPlante J-P, et al. Non-invasive technique for obtaining fluorescence excitation and emission spectra in vivo. Photochem Photobiol 1986;44(5):679–87.

[11] Anderson RR. Laser-tissue interactions. In: Goldman MP, Fitzpatrick RE, editors. Cutaneous laser surgery. 2nd edition. St. Louis (MO): Mosby; 1999. p. 1–18.

[12] Wilson BT. The physics of photodynamic therapy. Phys Med Biol 1986;31:327–60.

[13] Driver I, Lowdell CP, Ash DV. In vivo measurements of the optical interaction coefficients of human tumours. Phys Med Biol 1991;36:805–13.

[14] Frazier CC. Photodynamic therapy in dermatology. Int J Dermatol 1996;35:312–6.

[15] Lipson RL, Baldes EJ, Olsen AM. The use of a derivative of haematoporphyrin in tumour detection. J Natl Cancer Inst 1961;26:1.

[16] Lipson RL, Baldes EJ, Gray MJ. Hematopophyrin derivative for detection and management of cancer. Cancer 1967;20:2255.

[17] Dougherty TJ, Grindley GB, Fiel R, et al. Photoradiation therapy. II. Cure of animal tumors with hematoporphyrin and light. J Natl Cancer Inst 1975; 55(1):115–21.

[18] Dougherty TJ, Kaugman JE, Goldfarb A, et al. Photoradiation therapy for the treatment of malignant tumours. Cancer Res 1978;38:2628–35.

[19] McCaughan JS, Guy JT, Hawley P, et al. Hematoporphyrin-derivative and photoradiation therapy of malignant tumors. Lasers Surg Med 1983;3: 199–209.

[20] Szeimies RM, Hein R, Baumler W, et al. A possible new incoherent lamp for photodynamic treatment of superficial skin lesions. Acta Derm Venereol 1994; 74(2):117–9.

[21] Collins P, Robinson DJ, Stringer MR, et al. The variable response of plaque psoriasis after a single treatment with topical 5-aminolaevulinic acid photodynamic therapy. Br J Dermatol 1997;137:743–9.

[22] Morton CA, Whitehurst C, Moseley H, et al. Comparison of photodynamic therapy with cryotherapy in the treatment of Bowen's disease. Br J Dermatol 1996;135:766–71.

[23] Wolf P, Rieger E, Kerl H. Topical photodynamic therapy with endogenous porphyrins after application of 5-aminolevulinic acid. J Am Acad Dermatol 1993;28:17–21.

[24] Lui H, Salasche S, Kollias AT, et al. Photodynamic therapy of nonmelanoma skin cancer with topical aminolevulinic acid: a clinical histologic study. Arch Dermatol 1995;131:737–8.

[25] Orenstein A, Kostenich G, Tsur H, et al. Photodynamic therapy of human skin tumors using topical application of 5-aminolevulinic acid, DMSO and EDTA. Brault DJori GMoan J, et al, editors.

Photodynamic therapy of cancer II. Proc SPIE 1995; 2325:100–5.

[26] Fijan S, Honignsmann H, Ortel B. Photodynamic therapy of epithelial skin tumours using delta-aminolevulinic acid and desferrioxamine. Br J Dermatol 1995;133:282–8.

[27] Jeffes EW, McCullough JL, Weinstein GD, et al. Photodynamic therapy of actinic keratoses with topical aminolevulinic acid hydrochloride and fluorescent blue light. J Am Acad Dermatol 2001;45:96–104.

[28] Piacquadio DJ, Chen DM, Farber HF, et al. Photodynamic therapy with aminolevulinic acid topical solution and visible blue light in the treatment of multiple actinic keratoses of the face and scalp: investigator-blinded, phase 3, multicenter trials. Arch Dermatol 2004;140(1):41–6.

[29] Touma D, Yaar M, Whitehead S, et al. A trial of short incubation, broad-area photodynamic therapy for facial actinic keratoses and diffuse photodamage. Arch Dermatol 2004;140(1):33–40.

[30] Goldman MP, Boyce S. A single-center study of aminolevulinic acid and 417 nm photodynamic therapy in the treatment of moderate to severe acne vulgaris. J Drugs Dermatol 2003;2:393–6.

[31] Soler AM, Warloe T, Berner A, et al. A follow-up study of recurrence and cosmesis in completely responding superficial and nodular basal cell carcinomas treated with methyl 5-aminolaevulinate-based photodynamic therapy alone and with prior curettage. Br J Dermatol 2001;145:467–71.

[32] Rhodes LE, de Rie M, Enstrom Y, et al. Photodynamic therapy using topical methyl aminolevulinate vs. surgery for nodular basal cell carcinoma: results of a multicenter randomized prospective trial. Arch Dermatol 2004;140(1):17–23.

[33] Vincullo C, Elliot T, Francis D, et al. Photodynamic therapy with topical methyl aminolaevulinate for 'difficult-to-treat' basal cell carcinoma. Br J Dermatol 2005;152(4):765–72.

[34] Szeimes RM, Karrer S, Radakovic-Fijan S, et al. Photodynamic therapy using topical methyl 5-aminolevulinate compared with cryotherapy for actinic keratosis: a prospective, randomized study. J Am Acad Dermatol 2002;47(2):258–62.

[35] Parisar DM, Lowe NJ, Steward DM, et al. Photodynamic therapy with topical methyl aminolevulinate for actinic keratosis: results of a prospective randomized multicenter trial. J Am Acad Dermatol 2003;48:227–32.

[36] Lui H, Anderson RR. Photodynamic therapy in dermatology: recent developments. Dermatol Ther 1993;11(1):1–13.

[37] Bandieramonte G, Marchesini R, Melloni E, et al. Laser phototherapy following HpD administration in superficial neoplastic lesions. Tumori 1984;70: 327–34.

[38] Lui H, Hobbs L, Tope W, et al. Photodynamic therapy of multiple nonmelanoma skin cancers with verteporfin and red light-emitting diodes: two-year response and cosmetic outcomes. Arch Dermatol 2004;140(1):26–32.

[39] Warloe T, Peng Q, Moan J, et al. Photochemotherapy of multiple basal cell carcinoma with endogenous porphyrins induced by topical application of 5-aminolevulinic acid. In: Spinelli P, Fante MD, Marchesini R, editors. Photodynamic therapy and biomedical lasers. Amsterdam: Elsevier Science Publishers B.V.; 1992. p. 436–40.

[40] Warloe T, Peng Q, Heyerdahl H, et al. Photodynamic therapy with 5-aminolevulinic acid induced porphyrins and DMSO/EDTA for basal cell carcinoma. In: Cortese DA, editor. Fifth International Photodynamic Association Bienniel Meeting. Proc SPIE 1995;2371:226–35.

[41] Svanberg K, Andersson T, Killander D. Photodynamic therapy of human skin malignancies and laser-induced fluorescence diagnostics utilizing Photofrin and delta-aminolevulinic acid. In: Spinelli P, Fante MD, Marchesini R, editors. Photodynamic therapy and biomedical lasers. Amsterdam: Elsevier Science Publishers B.V.; 1992. p. 436–40.

[42] Svanberg K, Andersson T, Killander D, et al. Photodynamic therapy of non-melanoma malignant tumors of the skin using topical delta-aminolevulinic acid sensitization and laser irradiation. Br J Dermatol 1994;130:743–51.

[43] Calzavara-Pinton PG. Repetitive photodynamic therapy with topical delta-aminolaevulinic acid as an appropriate approach to the routine treatment of superficial non-melanoma skin tumors. J Photochem Photobiol B 1995;29:53–7.

[44] Jeffes EW, McCullough JL, Weinstein GD, et al. Photodynamic therapy of actinic keratoses with topical 5-aminolevulinic acid: a pilot dose-ranging study. Arch Dermatol 1997;133:727–32.

[45] Oseroff A, Shieh S, Frawley NP, et al. Treatment of diffuse basal cell carcinomas and basaloid follicular hamartomas in nevoid basal cell carcinoma syndrome by wide-area 5-aminolevulinic acid photodynamic therapy. Arch Dermatol 2004;141(1): 60–7.

[46] Hongcharu W, Taylor CR, Chang Y, et al. Topical ALA-photodynamic therapy for the treatment of acne vulgaris. J Invest Dermatol 2000;115:183–92.

[47] Pollock B, Turner D, Stringer MR, et al. Topical aminolaevulinic acid-photodynamic therapy for the treatment of acne vulgaris: a study of clinical efficacy and mechanism of action. Br J Dermatol 2004;151: 616–22.

[48] Papageorgiou P, Katsambas A, Chu A. Phototherapy with blue (415 nm) and red (660 nm) light in the treatment of acne vulgaris. Br J Dermatol 2000;142:973–8.

[49] Itoh Y, Ninomiya Y, Tajima S, et al. Photodynamic therapy for acne vulgaris with topical 5-aminolevulinic acid. Arch Dermatol 2000;136:1093–5.

[50] Itoh Y, Ninomiya Y, Tajima S, et al. Photodynamic therapy of acne vulgaris with topical delta

aminolevulinic acid and incoherent light in Japanese patients. Br J Dermatol 2001;144:575–9.

[51] Kennedy JC, Marcus SL, Pottier RH. Photodynamic therapy and photodiagnosis using endogenous photosensitization induced by 5-aminolevulinic acid: mechanisms and clinical results. J Clin Laser Med Surg 1996;14(5):289–304.

[52] Karrer S, Baumler W, Abels C, et al. Long-pulse dye laser for photodynamic therapy: investigations in vitro and in vivo. Lasers Surg Med 1999;25:51–9.

[53] Alam M, Dover JS. Treatment of photoaging with topical aminolevulinic acid and light. Skin Therapy Lett 2004;3(5):548–51.

[54] Dover JS, Bhatia AC, Stewart B, et al. Topical 5-aminolevulinic acid combined with intense pulsed light in the treatment of photoaging. Arch Dermatol 2005;141(10):1247–52.

[55] Ruiz-Rodriguez R, Sanz-Sanchez T, Cordoba S. Photodynamic photorejuvenation. Dermatol Surg 2002;28:742–4.

[56] Alexiades-Armenakas MR, Geronemus RG. Laser-mediated photodynamic therapy of actinic cheilitis. J Drugs Dermatol 2004;3(5):548–52.

[57] Von Tappeiner H, Jesionek A. [Therapeutic trials with fluorescent material]. Much Med Wochenschr 1903;47:2042–4 [in German].

[58] Von Tappeiner H, Jodlbauer A. [Regarding the photodynamic action of fluorescent material on protozoa and enzymes]. Dtsch Arch Kin Med 1904;80: 427–87 [in German].

[59] Lui H, Bissonnette R. Photodynamic therapy. In: Goldman M, Fitzpatrick R, editors. Cutaneous laser surgery. St. Louis (MO): Mosby; 1999. p. 437–58.

[60] Lee WL, Shalita AR, Poh-Fitzpatrick MB. Comparative studies of porphyrin production in *Propionibacterium acnes* and *Propionibacterium granulosum*. J Bacteriol 1978;133:811–5.

[61] Arakane K, Rya A, Hayashi C, et al. Singlet oxygen (1 delta g) generation from coproporphyrin in *Propionibacterium acnes* on irradiation. Biochem Biophys Res Commun 1996;223:578–82.

[62] Divaris DX, Kennedy JC, Pottier RH. Phototoxic damage to sebaceous glands and hair follicles of mice after systemic administration of 5-aminolevulinic acid correlates with localized protoporphyrin IX fluorescence. Am J Pathol 1990;136:891–7.

[63] Alexiades-Armenakas MR, Bernstein L, Chen J, et al. Laser-assisted photodynamic therapy of acne vulgaris and related conditions. Presented at the Amer Soc Las Surg Med Abstracts, Anaheim, California, April 2003.

[64] Alster TS, Tanzi EL. Photodynamic therapy with topical aminolevulinic acid and pulsed dye laser irradiation for sebaceous hyperplasia. J Drugs Dermatol 2003;2(5):501–4.

[65] Alexiades-Armenakas MR. Long-pulsed dye laser-mediated photodynamic therapy combined with topical therapy for mild to severe comedonal, inflammatory, or cystic acne. J Drugs Dermatol 2006;5(1):1–11.

[66] Seaton ED, Charakida A, Mouser PE, et al. Pulsed-dye laser treatment for inflammatory acne vulgaris: randomized controlled trial. Lancet 2003; 362(9393):1342.

[67] Orringer JS, Kang S, Hamilton T, et al. Treatment of acne vulgaris with a pulsed dye laser: a randomized controlled trial. JAMA 2004;291:2834–9.

[68] Hillemanns P, Untch M, Prove F, et al. Photodynamic therapy of vulvar lichen sclerosus with 5-aminolevulinic acid. Obstet Gynecol 1999;93(1):71–4.

[69] Alexiades-Armenakas MR. Laser-mediated photodynamic therapy of lichen sclerosus. J Drugs Dermatol 2004;3(6 Suppl):S25–7.

[70] Evans AV, Robson A, Barlow RJ, et al. Treatment of port wine stains with photodynamic therapy, using pulsed dye laser as a light source, compared with pulsed dye laser alone: a pilot study. Lasers Surg Med 2005;36(4):266–9.

[71] Kelly KM, Kimel S, Smith T, et al. Combined photodynamic and photothermal induced injury enhances damage to in vivo model blood vessels. Lasers Surg Med 2004;34(5):407–13.

[72] Smucler R, Jatsova E. Comparative study of aminolevulinic acid photodynamic therapy plus pulsed dye laser versus pulsed dye laser alone in treatment of viral warts. Photomed Laser Surg 2005;23(2):202–5.

DERMATOLOGIC
CLINICS

Dermatol Clin 25 (2007) 35–45

Aminolevulinic Acid-Photodynamic Therapy for Photorejuvenation

Pavan K. Nootheti, MD[a], Mitchel P. Goldman, MD[a,b],*

[a]*La Jolla Spa MD, 7630 Fay Avenue, La Jolla, CA 92037, USA*
[b]*University of California, San Diego, 9500 Gilman Drive, La Jolla, CA 92093, USA*

The concept of phototherapy is not a novel idea. Ancient civilizations in Egypt, India, and Greece used naturally occurring psoralens, found in various plants, for the treatment of pigmentary disorders [1,2]. 8-Methoxypsoralen was the main compound isolated from specific plants used to treat vitiligo and psoriasis. When light in the UVA range was able to be manufactured into UVA light bulbs, the concept of photochemotherapy was developed using topically applied 8-methoxypsoralen and UVA exposure. Photodynamic therapy (PDT) is a variation on phototherapy using a topically applied photosensitizing compound, 5-aminolevulinic acid (ALA), which is then activated by visible light irradiation for a predetermined period of time. PDT can also be used with photosensitizers that are taken systemically to achieve a greater area of photosensitivity.

PDT achieves its treatment response as ALA is activated through the use of visible light radiation. Singlet oxygen-free radicals are one of the free radicals produced that cause photo-oxidation of the target molecules, such as precancerous cells, tumor cells, sebaceous glands, vasculature, or superficial melanin. Two types of ALA are presently commercially available: Levulan (DUSA Pharmaceuticals, Wilmington, Massachusetts), which consists of 20% ALA solution with 48% ethanol, and 5-methylated ALA (MAL) in a cream base (Metvix, Photocure ASA, Oslo, Norway). MAL is available as a 16% strength cream in a 2-g tube. Levulan has been available in the United States since 1999 when it received approval by the US Food and Drug Administration for the treatment for actinic keratosis (AK). Metvix is available in Europe for the treatment of nonmelanoma skin cancer and AK and in the United States for the treatment of AK. ALA is left in place for absorption for varying time lengths based on the condition being treated and the form of ALA used. ALA esters, such as 5-aminolevulinic acid methyl ester and 5-aminolevulinic acid hexyl ester, have been compared with ALA in the effectiveness of skin penetration [3]. The stratum corneum is an important barrier for penetration of the different ALA chemicals. Tape-stripped skin increases the penetration by 100 to 200 times compared with normal skin. The skin penetration for both normal skin and tape-stripped skin is greatest for ALA and lowest for aminolevulinic hexyl ester into the skin.

After application of topical ALA, it is metabolized into the photosensitizer protoporphyrin IX (PpIX). Rapidly proliferating cells, such as tumor cells and sebaceous glands, accumulate PpIX. This is caused by the increased activity of porphobilinogen deaminase in tumor cells and the increased permeability of ALA in abnormal keratinocytes [4]. Nakaseko and coworkers [5] studied the histopathologic changes and involvement of apoptosis in tumor cell death after ALA-PDT using an excimer dye laser emitting 630-nm laser light. One hour after PDT, histopathologic findings revealed cells with eosinophilic cytoplasm and markedly stained nuclei in the basal layer of the epidermis, and some tumor cells showed vacuolation. The upper dermis had a scant infiltrate of lymphocytes and neutrophils.

* Corresponding author. La Jolla Spa MD, 7630 Fay Avenue, La Jolla, CA 92037.
E-mail address: mgoldman@spa-md.com (M.P. Goldman).

The same findings were even more evident in bi-opsy specimens taken 3 hours after PDT. One day after PDT and 3 days after, necrosis of all layers of the epidermis was noted in the tumor area. Seven days after PDT, the tumor cells in the epidermis had disappeared and regenerative thickening of the epidermis was noted. In the nor-mal areas of skin that did not have nuclear atypia in the epidermis, however, degeneration was detected.

Confocal spectral microscopy has been used to show the cellular events after ALA-PDT using a 488-nm argon-ion laser. Tsai and coworkers [6] reported that mitochondrial dysfunctions caused by ALA-PDT resulted in an increased cellular ad-hesion and reorganization of cytoskeletal compo-nents. It is possible that a combination of the previously mentioned mechanisms results in the clinical therapeutic benefits of photorejuvenation observed in ALA-PDT.

One advantage of PDT is its low incidence of serious side effects. The most common adverse effects include sensations of burning, stinging, or itching in the illuminated areas. Erythema and a degree of mild edema are usually noted in the treated areas and can be adequately controlled with a mild topical corticosteroid. Serious ad-verse events, such as ulcers, blisters, and necrosis, are usually rare and tend to be the result of excessive doses of illumination [4]. Photosensitiv-ity is one major undesirable side effect of PDT, sometimes lasting up to several days in locally treated areas. To avoid or limit photosensitivity, it is necessary to adhere to a strict regimen of total sun avoidance for 24 hours after the appli-cation of ALA.

Photodamage is not only unsightly leading to wrinkles, pigmentary unevenness and lentigines, telangiectasias, and textural changes, but it can also lead to precancerous conditions with the development of AK [7]. Numerous light sources have been documented to treat photodamage with PDT, such as blue light, red light, intense pulsed light (IPL), and the pulsed dye laser (PDL). Blue light sources use the maximum absorption peak of PpIX at 410 nm; however, the shorter wavelength of blue light provides less tis-sue penetration. Red light seeks to use one of the smaller absorption peaks of PpIX at 630 nm while maximizing tissue penetration with the lon-ger wavelengths. Several other light sources, such as broadband lamps, activate smaller peaks at 505, 540, and 580 nm. The choice of which light source to use for ALA-PDT depends on such fac-tors as the condition being treated, efficacy, and cost of use. Red light can penetrate 6 mm into the skin and is the desirable light source when deeper lesions are being treated. Light sources in the 400 to 500 nm range (blue light) are best used for superficial lesions because photon pene-tration is only up to 1 to 2 mm [8]. Fig. 1 demon-strates some of the various light sources used and their corresponding activating doses for PpIX; the x-axis represents the effective dose (joule per

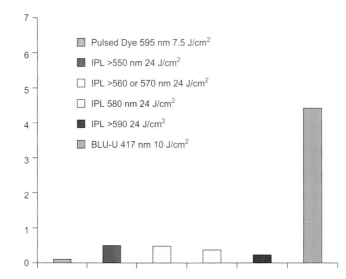

Fig. 1. Effective PpIX activating dose. (*From* Goldman MP, editor. Procedures in cosmetic dermatology series: photo-dynamic therapy. Philadelphia: Elsevier Saunders; 2005. p. 5.)

centimeter squared) and the y-axis represents the dose (joule per centimeter squared).

Photodynamic therapy with blue light

Photorejuvenation studies using the blue light source have been conducted by Goldman and coworkers [9], where a blue light source was used to illuminate the face after the topical application of ALA. Thirty-two patients with photodamage and AKs were treated with topical ALA for one session with a blue light source. ALA was applied to the whole face for 1 hour before the blue light treatment. AKs showed a 90% improvement and photorejuvenation parameters also showed a 72% improvement in skin texture and a 59% improvement in skin pigmentation (Fig. 2). Gold [10] documented that the use of a blue light source for ALA-PDT in the treatment of nonhyperkeratotic facial AKs also resulted in an improvement of skin elasticity and reduced skin thickening in patients with photodamaged skin. Touma and Gilchrest [11] studied the effectiveness of ALA and blue light illumination in the treatment of AK and diffuse photodamage. Eighteen patients

with facial nonhypertrophic AKs and mild to moderate facial photodamage were evaluated. ALA was applied from 1 to 3 hours with subsequent exposure to blue light. After 1- and 5-month intervals, there was a significant reduction in AKs and significant improvement in photodamage parameters, such as skin quality, fine wrinkling, and sallowness. Mottled pigmentation showed borderline improvement, but coarse wrinkling showed no improvement. Satisfaction was rated as good to excellent in more than 80% of the patients. It was also suggested in the study that the use of microdermabrasion just before application of ALA led to a more uniform and rapid penetration of ALA. In addition to proving the effectiveness of ALA-PDT using blue light, the study by Touma and Gilchrest [11] also emphasized the use of a 1-hour incubation for the ALA versus the traditional 14- to 18-hour ALA incubation times [12].

Photodynamic therapy with red light

The use of red light sources for ALA-PDT has also been documented to provide excellent cosmetic results. A study was performed to

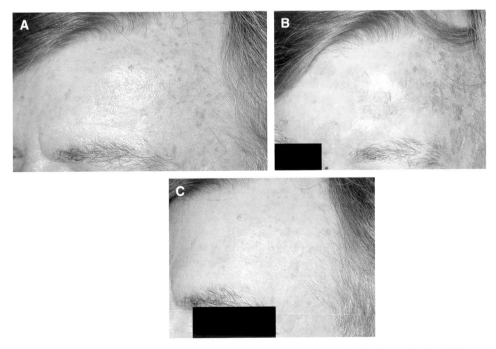

Fig. 2. (*A*) Lateral forehead of a 66-year-old man with numerous actinic keratosis. (*B*) One week after PDT treatment. Levulan ALA was applied to the entire area (not spot treatment) for 20 hours. The patient then was exposed to 1000 seconds of Blu-U treatment. Note crusting of all actinically damaged skin. (*C*) Appearance 1 year after treatment shows no evidence of actinically damaged skin or actinic keratosis. (*From* Nootheti PK, Goldman MP. Advances in photorejuvenation and the current status of photodynamic therapy. Expert Review of Dermatology 2006;1(1):51–61; with permission.)

investigate the photodynamic efficacy of irradiation with coherent light at wavelengths ranging
from 622 to 649 nm and it was suggested that
irradiation of human keratinocytes in vitro at 635
nm provided the best cell-killing effects [13]. Szeimies and coworkers [14] investigated PDT with
MAL in the treatment of AKs using a noncoherent
red light source (570–670 nm) versus cryotherapy.
They demonstrated that PDT using MAL is
a valuable treatment option for patients with
AK. PDT had a response rate similar to that of
cryotherapy, but the cosmetic results were superior with high patient satisfaction. In a similar
study, Pariser and coworkers [15] used a noncoherent red light source (570–670 nm) to illuminate
AK after application of MAL and found that it
was a safe and effective treatment of AKs, again
with excellent cosmetic results.

Photodynamic therapy with intense pulsed light

IPL is a light source that emits noncollimated,
noncoherent light with wavelengths in the range
of 500 to 1200 nm, which corresponds to the
visible light and near-infrared spectrum. Various
filters can be used to block certain wavelengths
below the cutoff point of the desired filter.
Although IPL alone has been proved effective in
the treatment of photodamage, the addition of
ALA to IPL treatment seems to be more effective
in treating photodamaged skin. Table 1 illustrates
the effective PpIX activating doses for various IPL
filter settings.

Ruiz-Rodriguez and coworkers [7] investigated
the treatment of photodamage and AKs using
ALA-PDT with IPL as the light source for photorejuvenation. Seventeen patients with various degrees of photodamage and AKs (38 AKs total)

underwent therapy with ALA-IPL. A total of
two treatments were performed with 1-month intervals and a follow-up evaluation at 3 months.
Thirty-three (87%) out of 38 AKs disappeared
and the treatment was well tolerated. Good cosmetic results were noted in the areas of wrinkling,
coarse skin texture, pigmentary changes, and
telangiectasias.

Avram and Goldman [16] evaluated the combined use of ALA-IPL for the treatment of photorejuvenation with one treatment session. A total
of 69% of the AKs responded to the use of
ALA-IPL and photorejuvenation parameters resulted in an improvement of 55% for telangiectasias, 48% for pigment irregularities, and 25% for
skin texture (Fig. 3).

Table 2 summarizes the recent peer-reviewed
reports of split-face ALA-PDT in the evaluation
of photorejuvenation. One of the split-face comparison studies was conducted by Alster and coworkers [17] to evaluate the effectiveness of the
combination ALA-IPL compared with IPL treatment alone. Ten patients received two treatments
with ALA-IPL on one side and IPL alone on
the contralateral side at 4-week intervals. Clinical
improvement scores were noted to be higher on
the side of the face treated with the combination
of ALA-IPL. They concluded that the combination of topical ALA plus IPL is safe and more effective than IPL alone for the treatment of facial
rejuvenation.

Marmur and coworkers [18] conducted a pilot
study to asses the ultrastructural changes seen after
ALA-IPL photorejuvenation. Seven adult subjects
were treated with a full-face IPL treatment; half of
the face received only IPL and the other half of the
face was pretreated with topical ALA before the
IPL treatment. Pretreatment and posttreatment
biopsies were reviewed by electron microscopic

Table 1
Effective PpIX-activating doses, updated for various IPL filter settings

	Dose (J/cm^2)	PAE coefficient	Effective dose (J/cm^2)	Dose to equal pulsed dye (J/cm^2)
Pulsed dye	7.5	0.0150	0.11	7.5
IPL (550 nm)	24	0.0207	0.50	5.4
IPL (560 or 570 nm)	24	0.0198	0.48	5.7
IPL (580 nm)	24	0.0152	0.37	7.4
IPL (590 nm)	24	0.0095	0.23	11.9
BLU-U	10	0.4425	4.42	0.3

Abbreviations: IPL, intense pulsed light; PAE, protoporphyrin activating exposure; PpIX, photosensitizer protoporphyrin IX.

From Goldman MP. Procedures in cosmetic dermatology series: photodynamic therapy. Philadelphia: Elsevier Saunders; 2005. p. 5.

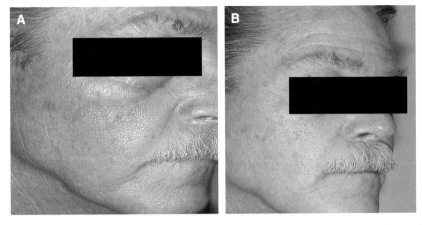

Fig. 3. (*A*) A 52-year-old man with extensive actinic damage and actinic keratosis of the face. (*B*) Six months after PDT treatment with a 1-hour application of Levulan ALA followed by IPL treatment with Lumenis One using a 560-nm cut-off filter, double pulse of 4 and 4 millisecond with a 10-millisecond delay at 18 J/cm², followed by 10 minute exposure with the Blu-U. (*From* Nootheti PK, Goldman MP. Advances in photorejuvenation and the current status of photodynamic therapy. Expert Review of Dermatology 2006;1(1):51–61; with permission.)

ultrastructural analysis for changes in collagen. A greater increase in type I collagen was noted in the subjects that were pretreated with topical ALA and treated with the IPL as opposed to the group treated with IPL alone. They concluded that the addition of ALA-PDT using IPL could be superior to IPL alone.

Dover and coworkers [19] also performed a randomized split-face study to assess the benefit of using ALA-PDT with IPL versus IPL alone. Twenty subjects had three split-face treatments 3 weeks apart with half of the face treated with ALA followed by IPL treatment and the other half treated with IPL alone. Two more additional full-face treatments were then performed to both sides of the face 3 weeks apart. A blinded investigator was used to evaluate the global photodamage, fine lines, mottled pigmentation, tactile roughness, and sallowness during the study.

They concluded that the pretreatment with ALA followed by IPL treatment resulted in greater improvement in global score for photoaging (80% versus 50%) and mottled pigmentation (95% versus 65%). Successful results were also noted for fine lines for the ALA-IPL side compared with the IPL side alone (55% versus 20%). Although tactile roughness and sallowness were noticeably better, pretreatment with ALA did not enhance the results of using ALA alone. It was important to note that both modes of treatment were well tolerated and that no significant differences in the side effect profiles were observed. They concluded that ALA-PDT using IPL for the management of photodamage provided results that were significantly better for global photodamage, mottled pigmentation, and fine lines in contrast to IPL alone without an increase in side effects. Fewer treatment sessions and better cosmetic

Table 2
Summary of recent peer-reviewed reports of 5-aminolevulinic acid-photodynamic therapy in actinic keratosis and measurement of photorejuvenation

Author	Year	Sensitizer and light source	Results
Alster et al	2005	ALA/IPL	ALA-IPL more effective than IPL
Marmur et al	2005	ALA/IPL	ALA-IPL could be superior to IPL Greater type I collagen increase with ALA-IPL
Dover et al	2005	ALA/IPL	Significantly better results and fewer treatment sessions with ALA-IPL than IPL
Gold et al	2005	ALA/IPL	ALA-IPL better than IPL

Abbreviations: ALA, 5-aminolevulinic acid; IPL, intense pulsed light.

results are provided with the ALA-IPL versus IPL alone.

Another split-face comparative study of ALA-PDT with IPL on one side and IPL alone on the other side was performed by Gold [20] to evaluate photorejuvenation. Subjects were treated with three IPL sessions at 1-month intervals. Results indicated that skin texture, mottled hyperpigmentation, facial telangiectases, and associated AK all showed better response to the side of the face treated with ALA-PDT. It could be clearly shown that ALA-IPL produced enhanced efficacy in photorejuvenation in addition to the effective treatment of AKs.

Photodynamic therapy with pulsed dye lasers

PDL as the light source for photorejuvenation with ALA has also been studied. Sterenborg and van Gemert [21] entered various numerical data on hematoporphyrin excitation and de-excitation into a mathematical model to test the effectiveness of PDT using different pulsed dye sources. It was noted that commonly used PDL using either a Copper vapor or a frequency doubled neodymium:yttrium-aluminum-garnet laser had a PDT effectiveness that was identical to a continuous wave laser source. Karrer and coworkers [22] investigated the efficacy of PDT both in vitro and in vivo using ALA with a long-pulse (1.5 millisecond) PDL. Human keratinocytes were incubated in ALA, then exposed to the long-pulse PDL at either 585, 595, or 600 nm, or an incoherent light source (580–740 nm). Twenty-four patients were treated with topical ALA and then exposed to the long-pulse PDL or an incoherent light source. They demonstrated that cytotoxic effects in vitro were maximized using the long-pulse PDL at 585 nm or the incoherent lamp. AKs treated on the forehead with ALA–long-pulse PDL achieved 79% clearing, whereas ALA combined with the incoherent lamp achieved 84% clearing. This study demonstrated both the in vitro and in vivo benefits of ALA-PDT using PDL.

Alexiades-Armenakas and Geronemus [23] found ALA-PDT with the 595 nm PDL was successful in treating both AKs and improving photorejuvenation. Their study included 2561 AKs on the face and scalp treated with ALA-PDT using a PDL. Clearance rates of 99.9% at 10 days, 98.4% at 2 months, and 90.1% at 4 months were noted. Lesions on the extremities and torso also showed improvement, although the rates were not as high as for the face and neck.

These results show the potential usefulness of a variety of lasers and light sources in the treatment of AK and in the improvement of photodamage and photorejuvenation using ALA-based PDT treatments. Beyond the active treatment of AKs, photodamage, nonmelanoma skin cancers, and beneficial cosmetic outcome for photorejuvenation, it is hoped that ALA may prevent or delay the onset of nonmelanoma skin cancers.

The use of ALA-PDT as a skin cancer prevention has to be considered experimental at present. Animal studies have been preformed by Sharfaei and coworkers [24] to examine this subject. Topical MAL-PDT was applied to half of the backs of hairless mice and the other side was treated with vehicle only and then exposed to UV radiation. It was concluded that topical MAL followed by light exposure under suberythematous conditions delayed the appearance of UV-induced skin tumors without increasing mortality or morbidity, and was able to show some benefit in preventing skin tumors. The underlying mechanism of action is still yet to be clarified. Some possible mechanisms include toxicity to the islands of mutated epidermal cells by some indirect phenomenon, a cytokine-mediated effect that delays tumor growth, reversal of UV-induced immunosuppression, or other specific antitumoral immune-mediated effects [25]. At present, some dermatologists are already using ALA-PDT as a skin cancer preventative mechanism.

Clinical technique

Because there are many different techniques to achieve similar results, there is no golden rule to follow with regards to the proper protocol. The following are general guidelines and principles for Levulan photodynamic photorejuvenation that could maximize treatment benefits for ALA-PDT that the authors use in their practice:

1. Patient washes their skin with soap and water.
2. Microdermabrasion with the Vibraderm is performed over the treated area.
3. The skin is then scrubbed vigorously with acetone on a 4 × 4 gauze.
4. Break the two glass ampules in the Kerastick as per instructions on the stick. Shake the stick for about 2 minutes. To see how the powder mixes with the solvent, remove the plastic Levulan Kerastick from the cardboard sleeve by pushing a pen or needle

driver into the end of the stick and the plastic sleeve extrudes from the cardboard sleeve.

5. Apply the contents on the area to be treated by painting the Levulan on the entire area. Do not worry about applying too much Levulan solution (recommend applying two coats of the solution). It is important to get close to the eyes, because it is apparent that the periorbital skin was not treated adequately if one fails to do this.

6. Allow the Levulan to incubate for 60 minutes on the skin indoors.

7. Wash the face before any treatment to remove the Levulan.

8. Activate the Levulan with the appropriate light source. The authors use an IPL followed by the BLU-U Light.

9. It is important to wash the face really well with soap and water after completing light treatments to remove any residual Levulan from the skin surface.

10. Warn the patient to remain out of direct sunlight for 24 hours. The authors recommend Niadyne cleanser and moisturizing night cream for 7 days after treatment. Ideally, patients should begin use of the Niadyne cream and cleanser 4 weeks before PDT treatment.

11. Patients are given Avene Thermal Spring Water spray to apply to their skin four to six times a day.

12. Repeat the treatment in 2 to 4 weeks. Increase incubation time if there was little reaction, and re-evaluate the skin preparation technique.

Multiple light sources can be used for ALA-PDT. Box 1 summarizes the most common parameters used in the authors' clinic. Appendices 1 to 5 consist of patient information and consent forms.

> ## Box 1. Parameters to activate Levulan for the most popular light sources
>
> **Lumenis One**: 560-filter, 18 J/cm^2, 4/4 with 10-msec delay, one pass.
>
> **Vasculight**: 560-filter; 30 J/cm^2, 2.4/4 with 10-msec delay, one pass or 35 J/cm^2 3–6 with 10-msec delay.
>
> **Quantum**: 560-filter, 26 J/cm^2, 2.4/4 with 10-msec delay, one pass or 30 J/cm^2 3–6 with 10-msec delay.
>
> **Aurora**: 16–22 J with a radiofrequency of 16–22 J, one pass.
>
> **Estelux**: 19–30 J at 20 msec, one pass.
>
> **V-Beam**: 10-mm spot, 7.5 J, 6-msec pulse width, two passes with 50% overlap.
>
> **V-Star**: 10-mm spot, 7.5 J, 40-msec pulse width, two passes with 50% overlap.
>
> **Clearlight**: 7 minutes under the light.
>
> **BLU-U**: 10 minutes under the light (Levulan can stay on the skin during the treatment)
>
> It is not necessary to adjust the parameters downward with an IPL when used with Levulan.

Management of adverse events

Most of the adverse events of ALA-PDT are related to patient discomfort and phototoxicity. Patient discomfort with complaints of burning, stinging, or itching can be handled with the proper patient education with what to expect and calming reassurance, because these symptoms usually improve on their own within a few hours after the treatment session. Phototoxic events are best prevented by using the proper parameters and the proper laser for the patient and with strict avoidance of the sun for 24 hours after the treatment session. If a phototoxic reaction does develop, the use of ice packs and topical corticosteroids usually suffices as treatment (Fig. 4). Cutaneous infections secondary to ALA-PDT therapy are usually low, but they can be managed with the appropriate topical antibacterial or antiviral medications. Following the precautions for patients with history of herpes simplex with the appropriate antivirals is important in preventing the reactivation of the virus (see Appendix 3).

Summary

A variety of lasers and light sources have been evaluated using ALA-PDT. These include blue light (405–420 nm); red light (635 nm); PDL (585 nm, 595 nm); and the IPL source (500–1200 nm). All of these devices have shown safety and efficacy in PDT and can be used in treating photodamaged skin. Physicians using these devices should be confident applying PDT in their patients.

The future of ALA-PDT is now. For many years, dermatologists have hoped that ALA-PDT would leave the laboratory setting and become part of everyday practice. Cosmetic improvements

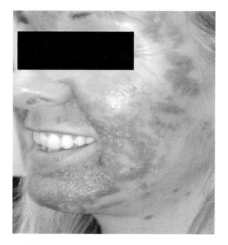

Fig. 4. This patient had a standard ALA-IPL treatment using a 1-hour incubation of Levulan ALA followed by IPL treatment. She then went horseback riding "at twilight" against medical advise and presented 24 hours later with an extensive sunburn. (*From* Nootheti PK, Goldman MP. Advances in photorejuvenation and the current status of photodynamic therapy. Expert Review of Dermatology 2006;1(1):51–61; with permission.)

have been shown in a variety of cutaneous concerns including photorejuvenation of photodamaged skin. Short-contact, full-face, broad-area ALA-PDT treatments make this therapy more practical for the dermatologic community[INSERT shppict]. Trials have shown that it is safe, efficacious, and relatively pain-free and without significant adverse effects. Clinicians should be ready for these new therapeutic approaches to common skin concerns and may rethink how dermatologists treat photodamaged skin, bridging closer the world of medical dermatology and cosmetic dermatologic surgery.

Appendix 1

Client Consent for Levulan® Photodynamic Treatment

Levulan® (Aminolevulinic acid 20%) is a naturally occurring photosensitizing compound which has been approved by the FDA to treat precancerous skin lesions called actinic keratosis. Levulan® is applied to the skin and subsequently "activated" by specific wavelengths of light. This process of activating Levulan® with light is termed Photodynamic Therapy. The purpose of activating the Levulan® is to improve the appearance and reduce acne rosacea, acne vulgaris, sebaceous

hyperplasia, decrease oiliness of the skin, and improve texture and smoothness by minimizing pore size. Any pre-cancerous lesions are also simultaneously treated. The improvement of these skin conditions (other than actinic keratosis) is considered an "off-label" use of Levulan®.

I understand that Levulan® will be applied to my skin for 30-60 minutes. Subsequently, the area will be treated with a specific wavelength of light to activate the Levulan®. Following my treatment, I must wash off any Levulan® on my skin. I understand that I should avoid direct sunlight for 24 hours following the treatment due to photosensitivity. I understand that I am not pregnant.

Anticipated side effects of Levulan® treatment include discomfort, burning, swelling, redness and possible skin peeling, especially in any areas of sun damaged skin and pre-cancers of the skin, as well as lightening or darkening of skin tone and spots, and possible hair removal. The peeling may last many days, and the redness for several weeks if I have an exuberant response to treatment.

I consent to the taking of photographs of my face before each treatment session. I understand that I may require several treatment sessions spaced 2-4 weeks apart to achieve optimal results.

I understand that medicine is not an exact science, and that there can be no guarantees of my results. I am aware that while some individuals have fabulous results, it is possible that these treatments will not work for me. I understand that alternative treatments include topical medications, oral medications, cryosurgery, excisional surgery, and doing nothing.

I have read the above information and understand it. My questions have been answered satisfactorily by the doctor and his staff. I accept the risks and complications of the procedure. By signing this consent form I agree to have one or more Levulan® treatments.

_____
Signature

_____
Print Name

_____

_____
Date Witness

Appendix 2

Therapy (PDT) Patient Guide

WHAT IS PHOTODYNAMIC THERAPY?

Photodynamic therapy (PDT) is a special treatment performed with a topical photosensitizing agent called Levulan® (5-aminolevulinic acid or ALA) activated with the correct wavelength of light. This is also known as "ALA/PDT treatment". These treatments remove sun damaged pre-cancerous zones and spots called actinic keratoses. Sun damage, fine lines, and blotchy pigmentation are also improved because of the positive effect of Levulan® and the light treatment. ALA/PDT treatment also has the unique ability to minimize pores and reduce oil glands, effectively treating stubborn acne vulgaris, acne rosacea, and improve the appearance of some acne scars.

HOW MUCH IMPROVEMENT CAN I EXPECT?

Patients with severe sun damaged skin manifested by actinic keratosis, texture, and tone changes including mottled pigmentation and skin laxity may see excellent results. You may also see improvement of large pores and pitted acne scars. Active acne can improve dramatically.

HOW MANY TREATMENTS WILL IT TAKE TO SEE THE "BEST RESULTS"?

To achieve maximum improvement of pre-cancerous (actinic keratoses) sun damage, skin tone and texture, a series of 2-3 treatments three to 4 weeks apart is most effective. Some patients with just actinic keratoses are happy with one treatment. More treatments can be done at periodic intervals in the future to maintain the rejuvenated appearance of the skin.

WHAT ARE THE DISADVANTAGES?

Following PDT, the treated areas can appear red with some peeling for 2-7 days. Some patients have an exuberant response to PDT, and experience marked redness of their skin. Temporary swelling of the lips and around your eyes can occur for a few days. Darker pigmented patches called liver spots can become temporarily darker and then peel off leaving normal skin. (This usually occurs over seven to ten days.) Repeat treatments may be necessary as medicine is not an exact science.

WHAT ARE THE ADVANTAGES?

1. Easier for patients than repeated topical liquid nitrogen, Efudex® (5-FU), or Aldara™ because the side effects are minimal, rapid healing, and only 1-3 treatments required.
2. The ALA/PDT treatment at our clinic is nearly painless verses liquid nitrogen, 5-FU and Aldara™.

3. Reduced scarring and improved cosmetic outcome compared with cautery, surgery and Efudex®. Liquid nitrogen can leave white spots on your skin.
4. Levulan® improves the whole facial area treated creating one color, texture, and tone rather than just spot treating with liquid nitrogen, cautery and surgery. In summary, PDT matches the "Ideal treatment" for actinic damage:
   • Well tolerated (essentially painless)
   • Easily performed by a specialty clinic environment
   • Non-invasive (no needles or surgery required)
   • Excellent cosmetic outcome (particularly in cosmetic sensitive areas of the face)

Appendix 3

Treatment Steps

1. Patients who have a history of recurring cold sores (Herpes simplex type I) should start oral Valtrex® 500 mg or Famvir® 250 mg tablets, one tablet twice daily for three days – starting this prescription the morning of your PDT treatment. The prescription for this product will be ordered for you.
2. Make sure your skin is clean and free of all make-up, moisturizers, and sunscreens. Bring a hat, sunglasses, and scarf when appropriate to the clinic.
3. Photography will be done by the staff before the Levulan® is applied.
4. You must sign a consent form.
5. An acetone scrub is performed. This will enhance the absorption of the Levulan® and give much more even uptake. In some patients microdermabrasion will also be performed immediately before the application of Levulan®.
6. Levulan® is applied topically to the whole area whole zone to be treated (such as the whole face, back of the hands, extensor part of the forearms).
7. The Levulan® is left on for 30-60 minutes before any light treatment.
8. The Levulan® is activated with the BLU-U® or IPL devise. This unique spectrum of light activates the Levulan® beginning with low energy levels.

9. Post-treatment instructions will be given to you to care for your improved skin.

Appendix 4

Home Care Instructions for Patients Following Photodynamic Skin Rejuvenation

Day of Treatment:

1. If you have any discomfort, begin applying ice packs to the treated areas. This will help keep the area cool and alleviate any discomfort, as well as help keep down any swelling. Swelling will be most evident around the eyes and is usually more prominent in the morning.
2. Remain indoors and avoid direct sunlight.
3. Spray on Avène Thermal Spring Water often.
4. Apply Niadyne™ moisturizing cream.
5. Take analgesics such as Advil® if necessary.

Day 2-7

1. You may begin applying make-up once any crusting has healed. The area may be slightly red for 1-2 weeks. If make-up is important to you, please see one of our estheticians for a complimentary consultation for DYG Mineral Make-up, which is all natural, inert, anti-inflammatory, and acts as a concealer with sunscreen. It is especially effective to mask redness.
2. The skin will feel dry and tightened. Niadyne™ moisturizer should be used daily.
3. Try to avoid direct sunlight for one week. Use a total block Zinc Oxide based sunscreen with a minimum SPF 30. We recommend Ti-Silc, Spa MD or Cool Clenz™.

Appendix 5

Levulan® Talking Points for Staff

1. Levulan® is all natural and produced by your body to make hemoglobin.
2. Levulan® is applied to your skin. There are no internal side effects.
3. Uptake of Levulan® is by abnormal cells. Levulan® targets these cells. (acne oil glands, pre-cancers).
4. Appropriate Light wavelength activates the Levulan®.

5. Your damaged skin then sheds leaving you with new, revitalized skin.

References

[1] Roelandts R. The history of photochemotherapy. Photodermatol Photoimmunol Photomed 1991;8:184–9.

[2] Pathak MA, Fitzpatrick TB. The evolution of photochemotherapy with psoralens and UVA (PUVA): 2000 BC to 1992 AD. J Photochem Photobiol B 1992;14:3–22.

[3] van den Akker JTHM, Holroyd JA, Vernon DI, et al. Comparative in vitro percutaneous penetration of 5-aminolevulinic acid and two of its esters through excised hairless mouse skin. Lasers Surg Med 2003;33:173–81.

[4] Kalka K, Merk H, Mukhtar H. Photodynamic therapy in dermatology. J Am Acad Dermatol 2000;42:389–416.

[5] Nakaseko H, Kobayashi M, Akita Y, et al. Histological changes and involvement of apoptosis after photodynamic therapy for actinic keratoses. Br J Dermatol 2003;148:122–7.

[6] Tsai JC, Wu CL, Chien HF, et al. Reorganization of cytoskeleton induced by 5-aminolevulinic acid-mediated photodynamic therapy and its correlation with mitochondrial dysfunction. Lasers Surg Med 2005;36:398–408.

[7] Ruiz-Rodriguez R, Sanz-Sanchez T, Cordoba S. Photodynamic photorejuvenation. Dermatol Surg 2002;28:742–4 [discussion: 744].

[8] Morton CA, Brown SB, Collins S, et al. Guidelines for topical photodynamic therapy: report of a workshop of the British Photodermatology group. Br J Dermatol 2002;146:552–67.

[9] Goldman MP, Atkin D, Kincad S. PDT/ALA in the treatment of actinic damage: real world experience. J Lasers Surg Med 2002;14:24.

[10] Gold MH. The evolving role of aminolevulinic acid hydrochloride with photodynamic therapy in photoaging. Cutis 2002;69(6 Suppl):8–13.

[11] Touma DJ, Gilchrest BA. Topical photodynamic therapy: a new tool in cosmetic dermatology. Semin Cutan Med Surg 2003;22:124–30.

[12] Touma D, Yaar M, Whitehead S, et al. A trial of short incubation, broad-area photodynamic therapy for facial actinic keratoses and diffuse photodamage. Arch Dermatol 2004;140:33–40.

[13] Szeimies RM, Abels C, Fritsch C, et al. Wavelength dependency of photodynamic effects after sensitization with 5-aminolevulinic acid in vitro and in vivo. J Invest Dermatol 1995;105:672–7.

[14] Szeimies RM, Karrer S, Radakovic-Fijan S, et al. Photodynamic therapy using topical methyl 5-aminolevulinate compared with cryotherapy for actinic keratosis: a prospective, randomized study. J Am Acad Dermatol 2002;47:258–62.

[15] Pariser DM, Lowe NJ, Stewart DM, et al. Photodynamic therapy with topical methyl aminolevulinate for actinic keratosis: results of a prospective randomized multicenter trial. J Am Acad Dermatol 2003;48:227–32.

[16] Avram D, Goldman MP. Effectiveness and safety of ALA-IPL in treating actinic keratoses and photodamage. J Drugs Dermatol 2004;3:36–9.

[17] Alster TS, Tanzi EL, Welsh EC. Photorejuvenation of facial skin with topical 20% 5-aminolevulinic acid and intense pulsed light treatment: a split-face comparison study. J Drugs Dermatol 2005;4:35–8.

[18] Marmur ES, Phelps R, Goldberg DJ. Ultrastructural changes seen after ALA-IPL photorejuvenation: a pilot study. J Cosmet Laser Ther 2005;7:21–4.

[19] Dover J, Arndt K, Bhatia A, et al. Adjunctive use of topical aminolevulinic acid with intense pulsed light in the treatment of photoaging. J Am Acad Dermatol 2005;52:795–803.

[20] Gold MH, Bradshaw VL, Boring MM, et al. Split-face comparison of photodynamic therapy with 5-aminolevulinic acid and intense pulsed light versus intense pulsed light alone for photo damage. Dermatol Surg 2006;32(6):795–801 [discussion 801–3].

[21] Sterenborg HJ, van Gemert MJ. Photodynamic therapy with pulsed light sources: a theoretical analysis. Phys Med Biol 1996;41:835–49.

[22] Karrer S, Baumler W, Abels C, et al. Long-pulse dye laser for photodynamic therapy: investigations in vitro and in vivo. Lasers Surg Med 1999;25:51–9.

[23] Alexiades-Armenakas MR, Geronemus RG. Laser mediated photodynamic therapy of actinic keratoses. Arch Dermatol 2003;139:1313–20.

[24] Sharfaei S, Juzenas P, Moon J, et al. Weekly topical application of methyl aminolevulinate followed by light exposure delays the appearance of UV-induced skin tumours in mice. Arch Dermatol Res 2002;294:237–42.

[25] Maari C, Bissonnette R. Treatment as prevention of skin cancer. In: Goldman MP, editor. Procedures in cosmetic dermatology series: photodynamic therapy. London: Elsevier; 2005. p. 55–63.

The Use of Photodynamic Therapy for Treatment of Acne Vulgaris

Mark S. Nestor, MD, PhD

Center for Cosmetic Enhancement, 2925 Aventura Boulevard, Suite 205, Aventura, FL 33180–3108, USA

Current topical and most oral therapies for acne vulgaris have limited efficacy, especially in moderate to severe cases. Photodynamic therapy (PDT) with 5-aminolevulinic acid (ALA) and recently methyl aminolevulinate has been shown to be a safe and effective modality for the treatment of acne vulgaris. Consensus guidelines suggest that 30 to 60 minutes is sufficient ALA contact time before photoactivation with blue light, red light, yellow light, broadband light, halogen, or pulsed dye laser (PDL) devices. An average of three treatments can yield significant long-term improvement.

Sebaceous glands

Sebaceous glands arise from hair follicles [1]. They are largest and most plentiful on the face, back, chest, and upper outer arms [2]. Undifferentiated sebocytes exist at the periphery of the gland and migrate toward the sebaceous duct as they mature. As they travel inward, sebocytes accumulate lipids, causing their volume to increase up to 150-fold [3]. When they reach the sebaceous duct, they disintegrate and discharge their contents into the duct as sebum [4].

Sebum consists of triglycerides (57%); wax esters (25%); squalene (12%); cholesterol esters (2%); and cholesterol (1%). As sebum flows through the follicular duct to the skin surface, bacterial lipases hydrolyze triglycerides to monoglycerides, diglycerides, and free fatty acids. In mammals, sebum maintains hydration of the hair and skin in the stratum corneum [4]. If sebum production becomes excessive, acne vulgaris may result.

The sebocyte migration time is approximately 14 days and the transit time of sebum in the follicular canals is approximately 14 hours [3]. The migration and ultimate rupture of sebocytes is regulated by androgens [5], primarily testosterone, which is converted by type I 5α-reductase enzyme to the more potent 5α-dihydrotestosterone [6]. Androgens also regulate the size of sebaceous glands. As circulating androgen levels increase during puberty, sebaceous glands become larger and more active, peak at 20 to 30 years of age, and become smaller and less active in later years [7].

Pilosebaceous unit

Sebaceous glands are part of the pilosebaceous unit (PSU), the target site of acne vulgaris. The PSUs also include a simple hair and a canal lined with stratified squamous epithelium [6]. The stratified epithelium is indirectly continuous with the surface of the epidermis [1]. In normal skin, desquamated cells are moved up the follicular canal by the flow of sebum [6]. As androgen levels rise during puberty, PSUs in sebaceous areas become sebaceous follicles in which sebaceous glands predominate over hair, which remains vellus. PSU disorders include acne vulgaris, hirsutism, and pattern alopecia [8].

PSUs normally harbor three groups of microorganisms: (1) aerobic micrococci and staphylococci, (2) semianaerobic *Propionibacterium acnes* and *Propionibacterium granulosum*, and (3) lipophilic yeasts [6]. *P acnes*, and to a lesser extent

Dr. Nestor has received research support and is a funded speaker, consultant, and physician advisory board member for Dusa Pharmaceuticals, Inc.

E-mail address: nestormd@admcorp.com

Staphylococcus epidermidis [9], have been implicated in acne vulgaris. Like the size and activity of sebaceous glands, the density of *P acnes* in skin increases at puberty, reaches a maximum in early adulthood, and remains constant until old age. *P acnes* colonization is highest in the face and scalp, where sebaceous glands are the most abundant [6].

Acne vulgaris

As one of the most prevalent skin diseases, acne vulgaris affects 80% to 85% of teenagers and may continue into adulthood. Acne vulgaris is the most frequent primary diagnosis in visits to dermatologists [10]. Although most often seen in adolescents, acne vulgaris may persist or even flare in the third and fourth decades of life, especially in women [11,12]. In the United States, the annual direct cost to treat acne vulgaris is estimated at more than $1 billion, which includes $100 for antiacne products sold over the counter [13,14].

The etiology of acne vulgaris is complex. Pathophysiology depends somewhat on clinical manifestations but overall is associated with four factors: (1) sebaceous gland hyperplasia with increased sebum production, (2) altered growth and differentiation of sebaceous follicles, (3) colonization of the follicle by *P acnes*, and (4) inflammation and immune response [15,16]. Although *P acnes* counts on the skin surface do not always correlate with severity of acne vulgaris, colony counts decline with clinical improvement. Clinical manifestations of acne vulgaris may be noninflammatory (comedones, open or closed); inflammatory (papules and pustules); and severely inflammatory (nodulocysts). Nodulocystic lesions often lead to scars [15,16].

Among the four factors of acne vulgaris development, altered growth and differentiation of sebaceous follicles and sebaceous gland hyperplasia in the PSU are the most important. Together they initiate the formation of microcomedos, the precursors of all acne vulgaris lesions [6,16]. Evidence suggests that comedogenesis of microcomedones occurs as abnormally desquamated keratin-filled cells (corneocytes), bacteria, and cell fragments accumulate in the PSU [16,17]. Microcomedones may undergo either comedogenesis or resolution, depending on environmental factors [18]. In patients with comedonal acne vulgaris, biopsy sections of clinically normal skin show histologic characteristics of microcomedones, suggesting that topical therapies should be applied to noninvolved skin and acne vulgaris lesions in acne-prone patients. Various types of comedones and their frequencies of occurrence have been described in detail [18].

Treatment of acne vulgaris

A variety of topical and oral agents are available for the treatment of acne vulgaris. Classical topical treatment includes cleansing (chemical and physical); antibiotic agents; benzoyl peroxide; vitamin A derivatives (retinoids); and acids (Table 1). Medications are applied daily and many are available without prescription. The goal of topical treatment is to prevent

Table 1
Medications for the treatment of acne vulgaris

Medication	Agents
Topical	
Retinoids	Tretinoin, adapalene, tazarotene, isotretinoin
Antibiotics	Clindamycin, tetracycline, doxycycline, lymecycline, minocycline, erythromycin, benzoyl peroxide, cotrimoxazole
Acids	Azelaic acid, salicylic acid
Oral	
Antibiotics	Tetracycline, doxycycline, lymecycline, minocycline, erythromycin, sulfamethoxazole-trimethoprim
Retinoids	Isotretinoin
Hormones	Estrogens; antiandrogens (cyproterone acetate, spironolactone, flutamide); oral contraceptives; glucocorticoids; gonadotropin-releasing hormone agonists (nafarelin, leuprolide, buserelin); 5α-reductase inhibitors

Data from Leyden JJ. A review of the use of combination therapies for the treatment of acne vulgaris. J Am Acad Dermatol 2003;49(3 Suppl):S200–10; Gollnick H, Cunliffe, Berson D, et al. Management of acne. a report from a Global Alliance to Improve Outcomes in Acne. J Am Acad Dermatol 2003;49(1 Suppl):S1–37.

the development of new lesions. Most dermatologists use combinations of topical products with or without oral antibiotics [6,15]. For example, combining benzoyl peroxide with topical antibiotics reduces the risk that resistant strains of *P acnes* develop [19]. Clindamycin and erythromycin are the most frequently used topical antibiotics in acne vulgaris [20].

Topical retinoid treatments for mild, mainly comedonal acne vulgaris are associated with a 38% to 71% reduction in inflammatory and noninflammatory lesion counts. Similarly, 50% to 70% reduction in total lesion count has been reported with combinations of topical retinoids, antibiotics, and benzoyl peroxide [14]. Alone or in combination, topical retinoids are considered first-line therapy for both comedonal and mild to moderate inflammatory acne vulgaris, minimizing the use of antibiotics [16] for acne vulgaris.

The use of topical agents is limited mainly by skin irritation, particularly in patients who require multiple topical agents. Benzoyl peroxide can bleach clothing and antibiotic use may cause resistance to develop [14].

Oral antibiotic agents, especially tetracycline and its derivatives, are indicated for moderate to severe inflammatory acne vulgaris; for treating lesions on the chest, shoulders, and back; and for patients with inflammatory acne vulgaris who have not responded to or cannot tolerate topical combinations [14,16]. Side effects of oral antibiotics include gastrointestinal upset (tetracycline, erythromycin); phototoxicity (doxycycline); hyperpigmentation (minocycline); and toxic epidermal necrolysis and allergic eruptions (trimethoprim-sulfamethoxazole) [14,16,21].

Oral isotretinoin has been a successful treatment of moderate to severe inflammatory acne vulgaris and nodulocystic acne vulgaris. One course of isotretinoin seems to be associated with approximately a 40% long-term clearance [22]. Side effects include birth defects, elevated results in liver function tests, and hypertriglyceridemia [14]. The use of isotretinoin has decreased significantly because of the government-mandated iPLEDGE program [23].

Hormones are useful in women if oral contraception is needed and in women not wanting to take isotretinoin for long periods. Hormone therapy is also appropriate for women with severe seborrhea, androgenic alopecia, acne tarda, hypergonadism, or seborrhea-acne vulgaris-hirsutism-alopecia syndrome [16]. Side effects include thromboembolism (oral contraceptives with estrogen) and menstrual irregularities or breast tenderness (spironolactone) [14].

Light and laser-based therapies

The need to minimize bacterial resistance to antibiotics and the side effects of topical and oral medications have led investigators to explore the well-known benefits of light on acne vulgaris lesions. In one of the first studies [24], the authors treated 30 patients with mild to moderate acne vulgaris with "full-spectrum" visible light, green light, and violet light three times weekly for 7 weeks. The results were evaluated by multiplying the numbers of comedones, papules, pustules, and infiltrates by severity indices before and after the series of treatments. Improvements were 14%, 22%, and 30% for full-spectrum, green, and violet light sources, respectively, and no side effects were reported. Improvement was greater on inflammatory pustules and infiltrates than on noninflammatory comedones. These observations led the authors to suspect that the therapeutic effect of the light was caused by eradication of *P acnes* by photodynamic destruction of porphyrins in the bacterial cells.

Among the four pathophysiologic factors [16] affecting the development of acne vulgaris, light had apparently affected only *P acnes* colonization. Phototherapy had not affected sebaceous gland hyperplasia with seborrhea; altered growth and differentiation of sebaceous follicles; and the inflammation process (although the response of inflammatory lesions to light was greater than that of noninflammatory lesions). The authors suggested that the benefit of phototherapy, although modest when used alone, might increase with more intense or more frequent treatments.

Three years later, Papageorgiou and colleagues [25] evaluated the use of 415-nm blue light and mixed blue and red light for the treatment of 107 patients with mild to moderate acne vulgaris. Patients were randomized into four treatment groups: (1) blue light; (2) mixed blue and red light; (3) cool white light; and (4) benzoyl peroxide (5%) cream. Patients were treated daily for 4 weeks and assessments were made every 4 weeks. At 12 weeks, inflammatory lesions of patients treated with mixed blue and red light improved 76% on average, which trended higher than improvements of patients treated with blue light, white light, or benzoyl peroxide alone. The 12-week mean improvement in comedones treated with mixed blue and red light was 58%, again trending higher than that of the other three treatments. The authors attributed the improvement with mixed blue and red light to the antibacterial effects of blue light and the anti-inflammatory effects of red light. (Red light had been shown in earlier studies to cause macrophages to release cytokines that ultimately influenced the inflammation, healing, and wound repair.) The mixed blue and red light treatment seemed to have affected two of the four pathogenic factors associated with acne vulgaris development.

Subsequent studies further explored blue light, lasers devices, and intense pulsed light for the treatment of acne vulgaris. Clinically, 420-nm blue light has been shown to reduce inflammatory acne vulgaris by 58% to >75% [26]. The mechanism for action of narrow band 420-nm light seems to be efficient killing of *P acnes* cells [27–30], one of the four pathogenic factors of acne vulgaris development.

The 1320- and 1450-nm yttrium-aluminum-garnet lasers have shown efficacy for the treatment of both inflammatory acne vulgaris and acne scarring [31–36] by destroying and shrinking sebaceous glands [37,38], another of the four pathogenic factors. One report describes the use of a long pulse 810-nm diode laser and indocyanine green dye selectively to target enlarged sebaceous glands rather than all sebaceous glands in an area [39]. The efficacy of the 585-nm PDL used alone is controversial [40,41] and an intense pulse light device combined with heat [42] has been shown to reduce both inflammatory and noninflammatory lesions. In the latter study, the authors suggested that the broadband light source (430–1100 nm) combined with heat addresses two of the four pathogenic factors: *P acnes* eradication by destruction of bacterial porphyrins (broadband light) and reduction of inflammation (heat combined with the red light). The KTP laser has also shown efficacy in the treatment of acne vulgaris [43].

Among the treatments discussed so far, retinoids address the altered keratinization patterns leading to impaction of the sebaceous follicle; antibiotics kill bacterial cells (some antibiotics also have anti-inflammatory effects); light therapies kill bacterial cells by porphyrin destruction; and some lasers shrink sebaceous glands. Each of these modalities addresses one or two of the four factors associated with acne vulgaris development. Oral isotretinoin, which reduces sebum secretion, the *P acnes* population, and inflammation, affects more pathogenic factors than any treatment

discussed so far. Isotretinoin also reduces comedo formation [44].

Photodynamic therapy

In PDT, a photosensitizer selectively accumulates in abnormal tissues and is activated by light in the presence of oxygen to initiate chemical reactions that destroy cells [45]. In 1990 Kennedy and colleagues [46] introduced the use of topical ALA photosensitizing agent for the treatment of cutaneous conditions by PDT.

In ALA-PDT, topical ALA penetrates the stratum corneum and accumulates in the epidermis and dermis of actinically damaged cells, solar keratoses, squamous cell carcinomas, basal cell carcinomas, and PSUs. Because ALA is the natural biosynthetic precursor of heme, it is converted to protoporphyrin IX (PpIX), a photosensitive compound. When the ALA-treated area is exposed to light of wavelengths in the absorption spectrum of PpIX, PpIX is activated to produce singlet oxygen, a metastable intermediate believed to be the cytotoxic agent in ALA-PDT [45,47,48]. In the United States, both ALA (Levulan Kerastick, Dusa Pharmaceuticals, Wilmington, Massachusetts) and methyl aminolevulinate (Metvix, PhotoCure ASA, Oslo, Norway) are approved by the Food and Drug Administration for the treatment of actinic keratoses of the face and scalp by PDT [45].

The foundation for the use of ALA-PDT in the treatment of acne vulgaris was provided by two groups of investigators [49,50]. Divaris and colleagues [49] injected ALA intraperitoneally into albino mice, and then showed that red fluorescence characteristic of PpIX was present in the sebaceous glands, and that fluorescence was weak in the epidermis and hair follicles. They then exposed the mice to activating light and studied the treated areas by light microscopy. The injection of ALA and subsequent exposure to light had destroyed sebaceous cells, produced focal epidermal necrosis with temporary acute inflammation, and caused reactive changes in keratinocytes. The severity and location of light-induced damage correlated with the intensity and location of red fluorescence and the fluorescence in the dermis was negligible. These results implied (but did not show) that the red fluorescence was caused by PpIX synthesized from the injected ALA, and that the treated sebaceous glands were destroyed a few hours after exposure to activating light.

Ten years later, Hongcharu and colleagues [50] reported a study in which they treated 22 subjects with mild to moderate acne vulgaris of the back. The investigators treated each patient at four sites. One site was treated with ALA (20%) and red light (550–700 nm); another site with red light alone; a third with ALA alone; and a fourth site was not treated. ALA was incubated for 3 hours under occlusion before exposure to red light. Eleven subjects were given a single treatment and the remaining 11 were treated four times. The authors studied protoporphyrin synthesis in PSUs, sebum excretion rate, autofluorescence from follicular bacteria, and histologic changes before and after treatment. Inflammatory acne vulgaris was cleared for 10 weeks and 20 weeks after one treatment and four treatments, respectively. Side effects included transient hyperpigmentation, superficial exfoliation, and crusting, all of which resolved without scar formation.

The significance of this study lies not only in the clinical improvement, but also in the demonstration of posttreatment reduction in sebum excretion rates, the suppression of bacterial porphyrin fluorescence associated with colonization of *P acnes* in sebaceous follicles, and in the damage done to sebaceous glands. These three effects, all pathogenic factors associated with acne vulgaris development, were observed only in the ALA-PDT–treated sites. After one ALA PDT treatment, sebum excretion rates decreased then gradually recovered. After multiple ALA PDT treatments, sebum excretion rates remained suppressed for at least 20 weeks. Compared with posttreatment fluorescence of the other three treatment sites, porphyrin fluorescence of *P acnes* was significantly reduced after a single ALA-PDT treatment and after four treatments. After a single treatment, sebaceous glands on the ALA-PDT–treated sites were reduced in size and sebocytes

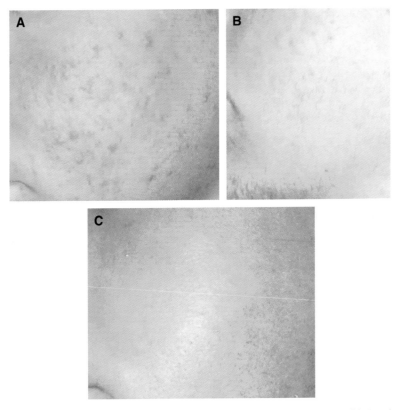

Fig. 1. (*A*) A 19-year-old man with moderate to severe acne before photodynamic therapy with 5-aminolevulinic acid. Patient received three treatments of photodynamic therapy with 5-aminolevulinic acid incubated 30 to 60 minutes. Activation was by pulsed dye laser (0.35-millsecond pulse duration, 2.6 J/cm² fluence). (*B*) One year after the final treatment. (*C*) Two years after the final treatment. (Courtesy of Mark S. Nestor, MD, PhD, Aventura, FL.)

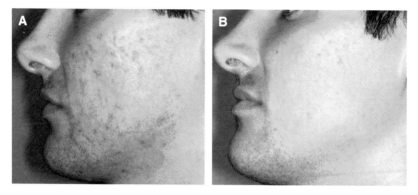

Fig. 2. (*A*) A 23-year-old man with moderate to severe acne before photodynamic therapy with 5-aminolevulinic acid. Patient received three treatments of photodynamic therapy with 5-aminolevulinic acid incubated 30 to 60 minutes. Activation was by pulsed dye laser (7-mm spot size, 0.5-millisecond pulse duration, 3.3–3.5 J/cm^2 fluence) followed by 420-nm narrowband blue light (5 minutes). (*B*) One year after the final treatment. (Courtesy of Mark S. Nestor, MD, PhD, Aventura, FL.)

were damaged compared with the other three treatment sites. Twenty weeks after a single ALA-PDT treatment, sebaceous glands were reduced in size, suggesting that the glands had started to recover. Twenty weeks after four ALA-PDT treatments, sebaceous glands were still partially damaged or completely destroyed, hair follicles were obliterated, and perifollicular fibrosis had occurred. Like oral isotretinoin, ALA-PDT with red light had affected three of the four pathogenic factors associated with acne vulgaris development.

Other PDT studies followed in which a variety of light sources (600–700-nm halogen [51], blue light [52,53], 635-nm red light [54,55], intense pulsed light [56,57], and long-pulsed PDL [58])

were used for activation in PDT. Wiegell and Wulf [55] used methyl aminolevulinate (3 hours incubation time) rather than ALA as a photosensitizing agent.

A recent study [58] evaluated the efficacy and safety of ALA-PDT with the long-pulsed PDL (595 nm) for the treatment of mild to severe cystic, inflammatory, and comedonal acne vulgaris of the face. All patients continued topical therapy during the study period. ALA incubation was 45 minutes. A mean of 2.9 treatments was required to achieve complete clearance in all 14 patients for a mean follow-up time of 6.4 months. Crusting, blistering, purpura, scarring, and dyspigmentation were not observed. This was the first study to show

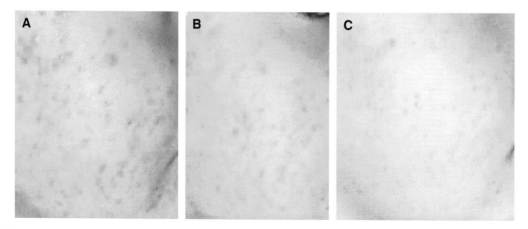

Fig. 3. (*A*) A 16-year-old girl with moderate to severe acne before photodynamic therapy with 5-aminolevulinic acid. Patient received three treatments of photodynamic therapy with 5-aminolevulinic acid incubated 30 minutes. Activation was by pulsed dye laser (0.35-millisecond pulse duration, 2.5 J/cm^2 fluence). (*B*) Three months after the final treatment. (*C*) One year after the final treatment. (Courtesy of Mark S. Nestor, MD, PhD, Aventura, FL.)

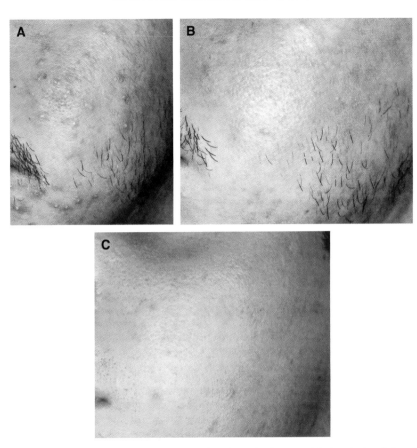

Fig. 4. (*A*) A 26-year-old man with severe acne before photodynamic therapy with 5-aminolevulinic acid. Patient received three treatments of photodynamic therapy with 5-aminolevulinic acid incubated 45 minutes. Activation was by continuous narrowband (yellow) light-emitting diode continuous light (16 minutes) followed by 420-nm narrowband blue light (5 minutes). (*B*) Six months after the final treatment. (*C*) Two years after the final treatment. (Courtesy of Mark S. Nestor, MD, PhD, Aventura, FL.)

complete clearance of mild to severe acne vulgaris with long-term follow-up by ALA-PDT with long-pulsed PDL.

Consensus conference for photodynamic therapy

A consensus conference was convened in June 2005 to review the use of PDT in cutaneous diseases [45]. Most of the discussion was restricted to ALA, the most extensively studied photosensitizing agent in the United States.

Regarding acne vulgaris, the following conclusions were stated:

> Consensus panel members agreed that ALA PDT provides (1) the best results when used to treat inflammatory and cystic acne and (2) modest clearance when used to treat comedonal acne vulgaris, although recent data shows that ALA

PDT was effective against comedonal acne vulgaris when the long-pulsed pulsed dye laser is used. They also agreed that (1) acneiform flares may occur after any treatment, including ALA PDT, and (2) although not supported by extensive documentation, PDL activation provides the best results in ALA PDT for acne vulgaris. One member (Dr. Nestor) stated that only PDL with ALA PDT has maintained clearance of acne vulgaris lesions for up to two years, even in patients resistant to other treatments.

Since the publication of the consensus guidelines, patients treated by the author have maintained acne lesion clearance when a continuous narrow-band (595-nm) yellow light light-emitting diode device (Gentlewaves LED Photomodulation, Light BioScience, LLC, Virginia Beach, Virginia) was used for photoactivation after ALA-PDT.

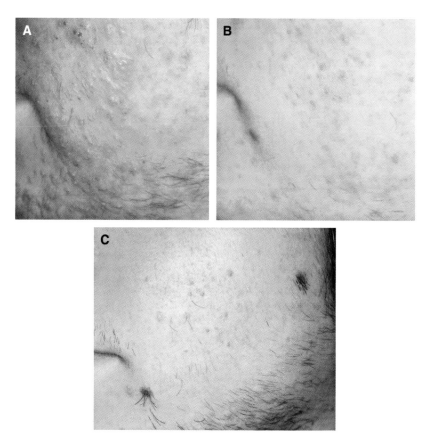

Fig. 5. (*A*) A 20-year-old man with severe acne before photodynamic therapy with 5-aminolevulinic acid. Patient received three treatments of photodynamic therapy with 5-aminolevulinic acid incubated 60 minutes. Activation was by continuous narrowband (yellow) light-emitting diode continuous light (16 minutes) followed by 420-nm narrowband blue light (5 minutes). (*B*) Eight weeks after the final treatment. (*C*) Six months after the final treatment. (Courtesy of Mark S. Nestor, MD, PhD, Aventura, FL.)

Panel members also suggested that physicians pretreat with microdermabrasion or scrubbing with acetone before applying ALA, allow ALA to remain in contact with skin for 30 to 60 minutes, and remove ALA before light treatment. Physicians should tell patients to expect mild to moderate redness, swelling, and desquamation after treatment. After treatment, panel members recommended applying titanium dioxide–zinc oxide to block UV light, instructing patients to avoid direct exposure to sun for 24 to 48 hours, and applying moisturizers as needed.

Treatment observations

In the author's experience, more than half of patients with moderate to severe acne vulgaris achieve virtual clearance with approximately three treatment sessions of ALA-PDT with either PDL

(V Star Pulsed Dye Laser, Cynosure, Westford, Massachusetts) or continuous-wave yellow light activation. Sessions are scheduled 2 to 3 weeks apart. With PDL activation, ALA is incubated 30 to 60 minutes before two laser passes (585-nm, short pulse, 7-mm spot size, 3.5 J/cm^2 fluence, 0.5-millisecond pulse duration) followed by 420-nm blue light treatment (8 minutes). Alternatively, patients receive a 16-minute treatment with continuous-wave yellow light. With both activation modalities, patients experience redness and peeling for 3 to 4 days. Preliminary experience with continuous red light activation (using red light-emitting diode panels on continuous mode (16 minutes of GentleWaves LED Photomodulation device) suggests that similar results can be obtained with this modality.

Improvement is clinically noticeable after the second treatment session. Three months after the first session, residual spotty erythema appears at the sites previously occupied by cystic lesions. Although initial flares occur in a few patients, overall acneiform eruptions are significantly reduced in most patients and clearance is achieved in approximately 50% of patients 6 months after the final treatment. Clearance persists for at least 1 year in most patients with 3.5 years as the longest follow-up time. Clinical examples are shown in Figs. 1–5.

In the author's hands, ALA-PDT has consistently provided significant improvement in moderate to severe papulopustular and nodulocystic acne vulgaris and significantly less improvement in mild and comedonal acne vulgaris. All side effects have been temporary. Redness and peeling have lasted up to 1 week in a few patients, many of whom failed to comply with instructions to avoid sun exposure for 24 to 48 hours after treatment. Two patients have experienced a pustular flare and three acquired secondary infection with gram-negative pathogens. Transient postinflammatory hyperpigmentation has occurred in a small percentage of patients.

Summary

ALA-PDT is a safe and effective modality for the treatment of mild to severe acne vulgaris. Like oral isotretinoin, ALA-PDT with red light affects three of the four pathogenic factors associated with acne vulgaris development. Consensus guidelines suggest that patients undergo pretreatment with microdermabrasion and that 30 to 60 minutes is sufficient ALA contact time before light or laser treatment. A recent study suggests that methyl aminolevulinate PDT may also be safe and effective, although short-contact methyl aminolevulinate (30–60 minutes) has not been studied. ALA-induced PpIX may be activated with blue light; red light; yellow light; broadband light (intense pulsed light); halogen (600–700 nm); and long-pulsed PDL. Side effects are limited to temporary redness and desquamation. Future studies are needed to refine further treatment parameters, provide guidance in selection of light sources, and identify potential subsets of patients most likely to benefit for PDT. Potential increased benefit may also be found in combining PDT with various topical and oral medications and light treatments.

References

[1] Montagna W. An introduction to sebaceous glands. J Invest Dermatol 1974;62:120–3.

[2] Habif TP. Clinical dermatology: a color guide to diagnosis and therapy. 4th edition. New York: Mosby; 2004.

[3] Downing DT, Steward ME, Strauss JS. Changes in sebum secretion and the sebaceous gland. Dermatol Clin 1986;4:419–23.

[4] Leyden JJ. New understandings of the pathogenesis of acne. J Am Acad Dermatol 1995;32(5 Pt 3): S15–25.

[5] Cunliffe WJ, Simpson NB. Disorders of the sebaceous gland. In: Champion RH, Burton JL, Burns DA, et al, editors. Textbook of dermatology. 6th edition. Oxford: Blackwell Science; 1998. p. 1927–84.

[6] Gollnick H. Current concepts of the pathogenesis of acne: implications for drug treatment. Drugs 2003; 63:1579–96.

[7] Hogan D, Jones RW, Mason SH. Sebaceous hyperplasia. Available at: http://www.emedicine.com/derm/topic395.htm. Accessed April 14, 2006.

[8] Deplewski D, Rosenfield RL. Role of hormones in pilosebaceous unit development. Endocr Rev 2000; 21:363–92.

[9] Nishijima S, Kurokawa I, Katoh N, et al. The bacteriology of acne vulgaris and antimicrobial susceptibility of *Propionibacterium acnes* and *Staphylococcus epidermidis* isolated from acne lesions. J Dermatol 2000;27:318–23.

[10] Stern RS. Dermatologists and office-based care of dermatologic disease in the 21st century. J Investig Dermatol Symp Proc 2004;9:126–30.

[11] White GM. Recent findings in the epidemiologic evidence, classification, and subtypes of acne vulgaris. J Am Acad Dermatol 1998;39(2 Pt 3):S34–7.

[12] O'Loughlin M. Acne in the adult female. Australas J Dermatol 1964;14:218–22.

[13] Management of acne: summary, evidence/report technology assessment. No. 17. Rockville (MD): Agency for Healthcare Research and Quality, AHRQ publication no. 01–E018; 2001.

[14] James WD. Clinical practice: acne. N Engl J Med 2005;352:1463–72.

[15] Leyden JJ. A review of the use of combination therapies for the treatment of acne vulgaris. J Am Acad Dermatol 2003;49(3 Suppl):S200–10.

[16] Gollnick H, Cunliffe W, Berson D, et al. Management of acne: a report from a Global Alliance to Improve Outcomes in Acne. J Am Acad Dermatol 2003;49(1 Suppl):S1–37.

[17] Holmes RL, Williams M, Cunliffe WJ. Pilo-sebaceous duct obstruction and acne. Br J Dermatol 1972;87:327–32.

[18] Cunliffe WJ, Holland DB, Clark SM, et al. Comedogenesis: some new aetiological, clinical and therapeutic strategies. Br J Dermatol 2000;142: 1084–91.

[19] Eady EA, Bojar RA, Jones CE, et al. The effects of acne treatment with a combination of benzoyl peroxide and erythromycin on skin carriage of

erythromycin-resistant propionibacteria. Br J Dermatol 1996;134:107–13.

[20] Johnson BA, Nunley JR. Topical therapy for acne vulgaris. How do you choose the best drug for each patient? Postgrad Med 2000;107:69–70, 73–6, 79–80.

[21] Meynadier J, Allirezai M. Systemic antibiotics for acne. Dermatology 1998;196:135–9.

[22] White GM. Acne therapy. Adv Dermatol 1999;14:29–58.

[23] Kilgore C. Prescribing down as derms' iPLEDGE angst continues: FDA chief hears complaints from senators. Skin and Allergy News 2006;37:1, 26–7.

[24] Sigurdsson V, Knulst A, van Weelden H. Phototherapy of acne vulgaris with visible light. Dermatology 1997;194:256–60.

[25] Papageorgiou P, Katsambas A, Chu A. Phototherapy with blue (415 nm) and red (660 nm) light in the treatment of acne vulgaris. Br J Dermatol 2000;142:973–8.

[26] Gold MH. The utilization of ALA PDT and a new photoclearing device for the treatment of severe inflammatory acne vulgaris: results of an initial clinical trial. J Lasers Surg Med 2003;15:S46.

[27] Omi T, Bjerring P, Sato S, et al. 420 nm intense continuous light therapy for acne. J Cosmet Laser Ther 2004;6:156–62.

[28] Tzung TY, Wu KH, Huang ML. Blue light phototherapy in the treatment of acne. Photodermatol Photoimmunol Photomed 2004;20:266–9.

[29] Elman M, Slatkine M, Harth Y. The effective treatment of acne vulgaris by a high-intensity, narrow band 405–420 nm light source. J Cosmet Laser Ther 2003;5:111–7.

[30] Kawada A, Aragane Y, Kameyama H, et al. Acne phototherapy with a high-intensity, enhanced, narrow-band, blue light source: an open study and in vitro investigation. J Dermatol Sci 2002;30:129–35.

[31] Friedman P, Jih M, Kimyai-Asadi A, et al. Treatment of inflammatory facial acne vulgaris with the 1450-nm diode laser: a pilot study. Dermatol Surg 2004;30:147–51.

[32] Wang S, Counters J, Flor M, et al. Treatment of inflammatory facial acne with the 1,450 nm diode laser alone versus microdermabrasion plus the 1,450 nm laser: a randomized, split-face trial. Dermatol Surg 2006;32:249–55.

[33] Jih MH, Friedman PM, Goldberg LH, et al. The 1450-nm diode laser for facial inflammatory acne vulgaris: dose-response and 12-month follow-up study. J Am Acad Dermatol 2006;55:80–7.

[34] Fulchiero GH Jr, Parham-Vetter PC, Obagi S. Subcision and 1320-nm Nd:YAG nonablative laser resurfacing for the treatment of acne scars: a simultaneous split-face single patient trial. Dermatol Surg 2004;30:1356–9.

[35] Sadick NS, Schecter AK. A preliminary study of utilization of the 1320-nm Nd:YAG laser for the treatment of acne scarring. Dermatol Surg 2004;30:995–1000.

[36] Rogachefsky AS, Hussain M, Goldberg DJ. Atrophic and a mixed pattern of acne scars improved with a 1320-nm Nd:YAG laser. Dermatol Surg 2003;29:904–8.

[37] Paithankar D, Ross E, Saleh B, et al. Acne treatment with a 1,450 nm wavelength laser and cryogen spray cooling. Lasers Surg Med 2002;31:106–14.

[38] Elman M, Lebzelter J. Light therapy in the treatment of acne vulgaris. Dermatol Surg 2004;30:139–46.

[39] Lloyd J, Mirkov M. Selective photothermolysis of the sebaceous glands for acne treatment. Lasers Surg Med 2002;31:115–20.

[40] Seaton E, Charakida A, Mouser P, et al. Pulsed-dye laser treatment for inflammatory acne vulgaris: randomised controlled trial. Lancet 2003;362:1347–52.

[41] Orringer J, Kang S, Hamilton T, et al. Treatment of acne vulgaris with a pulsed dye laser: a randomized controlled trial. JAMA 2004;291:2834–9.

[42] Elman M, Lask G. The role of pulsed light and heat energy (LHE) in acne clearance. J Cosmet Laser Ther 2004;6:91–5.

[43] Baugh W, Kucaba W. Nonablative phototherapy for acne vulgaris using the KTP 532 nm laser. Dermatol Surg 2005;31:1290–6.

[44] Webster GF. Laser treatment of acne. Lancet 2003;362:1342.

[45] Nestor M, Gold M, Kauvar A, et al. The use of photodynamic therapy in dermatology: results of a consensus conference. J Drugs Dermatol 2006;5:140–54.

[46] Kennedy JC, Pottier RH, Pross DC. Photodynamic therapy with endogenous protoporphyrin IX: basic principles and present clinical experience. J Photochem Photobiol B 1990;6:143–8.

[47] Weishaupt KR, Gomer CJ, Dougherty TJ. Identification of singlet oxygen as the cytotoxic agent in photoinactivation of a murine tumor. Cancer Res 1976;36(7 Pt 1):2326–9.

[48] Niedre MJ, Yu CS, Patterson MS, et al. Singlet oxygen luminescence as an in vivo photodynamic therapy dose metric: validation in normal mouse skin with topical amino-levulinic acid. Br J Cancer 2005;92:298–304.

[49] Divaris DX, Kennedy JC, Pottier RH. Phototoxic damage to sebaceous glands and hair follicles of mice after systemic administration of 5-aminolevulinic acid correlates with localized protoporphyrin IX fluorescence. Am J Pathol 1990;136:891–7.

[50] Hongcharu W, Taylor C, Chang Y, et al. Topical ALA-photodynamic therapy for the treatment of acne vulgaris. J Invest Dermatol 2000;115:183–92.

[51] Itoh Y, Ninomiya Y, Tajima S, et al. Photodynamic therapy of acne vulgaris with topical delta-aminolaevulinic acid and incoherent light in Japanese patients. Br J Dermatol 2001;144:575–9.

[52] Goldman M, Boyce S. A single-center study of aminolevulinic acid and 417 NM photodynamic therapy in the treatment of moderate to severe acne vulgaris. J Drugs Dermatol 2003;2:393–6.

[53] Taub A. Photodynamic therapy for the treatment of acne: a pilot study. J Drugs Dermatol 2004; 3(6 Suppl):S10–4.

[54] Pollock B, Turner D, Stringer M, et al. Topical aminolaevulinic acid-photodynamic therapy for the treatment of acne vulgaris: a study of clinical efficacy and mechanism of action. Br J Dermatol 2004;151: 616–22.

[55] Wiegell SR, Wulf HC. Photodynamic therapy of acne vulgaris using methyl aminolaevulinate: a blinded, randomized, controlled trial. Br J Dermatol 2006;154:969–76.

[56] Gold M, Bradshaw V, Boring M, et al. The use of a novel intense pulsed light and heat source and ALA-PDT in the treatment of moderate to severe inflammatory acne vulgaris. J Drugs Dermatol 2004; 3(6 Suppl):S15–9.

[57] Santos M, Belo V, Santos G. Effectiveness of photodynamic therapy with topical 5-aminolevulinic acid and intense pulsed light versus intense pulsed light alone in the treatment of acne vulgaris: comparative study. Dermatol Surg 2005;31: 910–5.

[58] Alexiades-Armenakas M. Long-pulsed dye laser-mediated photodynamic therapy combined with topical therapy for mild to severe comedonal, inflammatory, or cystic acne. J Drugs Dermatol 2006;5:45–55.

DERMATOLOGIC
CLINICS

Dermatol Clin 25 (2007) 59–65

Aminolevulinic Acid Photodynamic Therapy for Sebaceous Gland Hyperplasia

Donald F. Richey, MD

North Valley Dermatology Center, 251 Cohasset Road, Suite 240, Chico, CA 95926, USA

The sebaceous glands are most abundant and largest on the face, back, chest, and upper outer arms [1]. They are aggregates of different-sized, acini that arise from hair follicles. Each acinus empties into a network of ducts that is continuous with the pilary canal. As cells of the sebaceous gland (sebocytes) mature, they move from the periphery of the gland to the central excretory sebaceous duct. They accumulate lipid until they reach the sebaceous duct where they rupture, release their lipid-laden cytoplasm, and die [2,3]. The dead cellular materials combine with desquamating cells of the lower hair follicle and travel to the skin surface as sebum [1].

The activity and size of sebaceous glands vary with age and levels of circulating androgens. Although large at birth, sebaceous glands become smaller during childhood; however; they become larger and more active during puberty as androgen production increases. Sebaceous gland size and activity peak at age 20 to 30 years. In later years, sebaceous cell turnover decreases as androgen levels decrease [2].

Sebaceous hyperplasia

When cellular turnover is reduced, undifferentiated sebaceous cells begin to crowd the glandular lobules, which results in sebaceous hyperplasia (SH). The glands enlarge and become conspicuous in areas such as the face, where they are numerous. Although these hyperplastic glands may be 10 times as large as normal glands, they secrete only small amounts of sebum because their cells are small and undifferentiated; they contain only small quantities of lipid and their nuclei are enlarged [2]. These primitive cells also move more slowly toward the sebaceous duct than do their counterparts in normal glands [4–6].

SH lesions are benign and occur most frequently in adults and the aged. They may occur at earlier ages in immunosuppression with cyclosporin [7,8], familial cases [9], Muir-Torre syndrome [10,11], pachydermoperiostosis [12,13], and in association with X-chromosomal hypohidrotic ectodermal dysplasia [14]. SH lesions at puberty [15,16] and "giant" lesions [17–19] also have been reported. Patients (especially elderly ones) seek treatment for cosmetic reasons [20].

SH lesions are round, yellow papules 2 to 3 mm in size and have a central depression resulting from a dilated excretion duct [21,22]. SH lesions may occur singly or as multiple lesions, with up to 50 present on the nose, forehead, and cheeks [6,23]. The cause of SH is not known in most cases, although systemic corticosteroids [7,24] and hemodialysis [25] have been implicated [22]. Differentiation of SH lesions from those of sebaceous nevus, sebaceous adenoma, sebaceous epithelioma, basal cell carcinoma, molluscum contagiosum, and xanthoma is important [21], and sometimes requires biopsy [26].

SH has been treated by a variety of methods. This article summarizes the advantages and disadvantages of various therapies, and describes how photodynamic therapy (PDT) with 5-aminolevulinic acid (ALA) has emerged as a safe and effective option for the treatment of SH.

Dr. Richey is a consultant and funded speaker for Dusa Pharmaceuticals, Inc. He has no financial interest in products developed by Dusa Pharmaceuticals.

E-mail address: drichey132@aol.com

Current therapies

SH has been treated with isotretinoin [9,27–29], surgical excision, topical chemicals, cryotherapy [30], bichloroacetic acid [31], electrodessication and curettage, intralesional desiccation [32], and lasers [22,23,33–36].

During the 1980s, researchers found that oral isotretinoin could clear multiple lesions within 2 to 6 weeks, but lesions recurred when isotretinoin was discontinued [9,28,29]. More recently, isotretinoin use has been made cumbersome by US Food and Drug Administration (FDA) regulations that limit its use. Destructive modalities, such as cryotherapy, surgical excision, cauterization, topical agents, and curettage with electrodessication, have a high risk for scarring, dyspigmentation, intra- and postoperative bleeding, and lesion recurrence [23,37]. With cryotherapy, each lesion must be treated individually [30], which renders this procedure time consuming and tedious when lesions are numerous. With bichloroacetic acid [31], small atrophic scars and prolonged stinging occur; care must be taken to avoid contact with normal skin (especially the eyes) during treatment.

The argon, CO_2, 585-nm pulsed dye, and 1450-nm diode laser devices have been used to treat SH lesions. Landthaler and colleagues [33] obtained "preliminary promising results" in five patients when they treated SH lesions with blue and green argon laser energy. They gave multiple treatments spaced 3 weeks apart. Treatment settings were 2.6 W power, 0.3 seconds pulse duration, 2-mm spot size, 83 W/cm^2, and 25 J/cm^2. The investigators attributed efficacy to the laser's nonspecific coagulation effect.

Marsili and colleagues [34] used a focused CO_2 laser beam to treat the nodules of a hemangioma that was associated with rhinophyma. In this study, SH lesions were present on the angioma as an overgrowth of soft tissue.

Schonermark and colleagues [22] used a 585-nm pulsed dye laser (PDL; a "vascular" laser) to treat a single SH lesion on the forehead of one patient and multiple SH lesions on the forehead of another. After three sessions, the single lesion resolved without recurrence or scarring after 13 months. The multiple lesions of the other patient resolved without recurrence or scarring for at least 9 months. The investigators attributed the absence of posttreatment scars to selective photothermolysis, which damages only the target tissue without harming the surrounding tissue. The efficacy was attributed to selective destruction of blood vessels (the target tissue) supplying the sebaceous gland.

Two years, later Gonzalez and colleagues [35], in their search to explain the PDL's efficacy in SH, used in vivo confocal imaging to observe the histologic changes in the vascular components of the SH lesions before and after PDL treatment. One year later, Aghassi and colleagues [23] used real-time confocal scanning laser microscopy to study the blood vessels surrounding the sebaceous duct and their coagulation resulting from 585-nm PDL treatment.

Because the 1450-nm diode laser device has an indication for the treatment of acne of the back, No and colleagues [36] evaluated the efficacy and safety of this device in the treatment of more than 330 SH lesions of 10 patients. Patients were treated one to five times at 5- to 6-week intervals. After several treatments, 84% of lesions had shrunk more than 50% and 70% had shrunk more than 75%. One atrophic scar and one case of temporary hyperpigmentation were reported. Because the target of the 1450-nm laser is water, the investigators speculated that the SH glands probably were destroyed by heat, the mechanism by which this same laser destroys acne lesions.

Aminolevulinic acid photodynamic therapy

PDT with ALA is a safe and effective treatment of actinic keratosis (AK), photodamage, acne vulgaris, and sebaceous hyperplasia. Success in treating less common conditions, including superficial nonmelanoma skin cancers, also has been reported [38–40].

PDT with topical ALA was introduced in the early 1990s by Kennedy and colleagues [41,42], who evaluated the technique for the treatment of AK, superficial basal cell carcinoma, squamous cell carcinoma, and metastatic carcinoma of the breast. Their encouraging results motivated investigators to apply ALA-PDT to other skin conditions and to vary treatment parameters, such as ALA incubation time and the light source. ALA is applied to the skin and allowed to incubate for 30 minutes or longer, depending on the condition being treated. ALA penetrates abnormal tissue more rapidly than it enters normal tissue, thus conferring selectivity to the procedure [41]. As ALA enters tissue cells, it is converted to protoporphyrin IX (PpIX). In this application, ALA acts as a photosensitizing agent because, in its conversion to photosensitive PpIX, ALA photosensitizes the target tissue. When sufficient ALA has entered target tissue, residual ALA is wiped away and the treated area is exposed to wavelengths of light in the absorption spectrum of PpIX. PpIX, in the presence of molecular oxygen and light, is activated to produce singlet oxygen, an unstable intermediate that destroys the cells in which it is produced [41,42].

In 1999, the FDA cleared Levulan Kerastick (Dusa Pharmaceuticals, Inc., Wilmington, Massachusetts) as ALA for the treatment of multiple AKs on the scalp and head, and the BLU-U Blue Light Photodynamic Therapy Illuminator (Dusa Pharmaceuticals, Inc.) for the treatment of AK. The BLU-U also is FDA cleared for the treatment of moderate inflammatory acne vulgaris. Levulan is the only FDA-cleared preparation of ALA that is available in the United States at the time of this writing.

The basic science

PpIX also accumulates in pilosebaceous units and is metabolized to PpIX [42–45], a finding that led to evaluations of ALA-PDT for the treatment of acne vulgaris [45–51] and SH [20,40,52,53].

The study of Divaris and colleagues [43] was undertaken to identify areas of albino mouse skin that would acquire PpIX-associated fluorescence and undergo phototoxic damage when exposed to activating light after injection of ALA. Intraperitoneal injection of ALA resulted in the development of intense red fluorescence (due to PpIX) in the sebaceous glands and little or no fluorescence in the epidermis, hair follicle, dermis, blood vessels, and ear cartilage of mice. Subsequent exposure of the ALA-injected mice to activating light resulted in destruction of sebaceous cells. In general, phototoxic damage correlated well with the location and intensity of red fluorescence; areas of skin exposed to light appeared to recover well from the treatment. This study showed that ALA selectively accumulates in sebaceous glands after intraperitoneal injection and subsequent irradiation with red light destroyed sebaceous glands in albino mice.

Encouraged by these results and the work of Kennedy and Pottier [42], Hongcharu and colleagues [45] treated 22 patients who had mild to moderate acne (on the back) with ALA-PDT to determine if this new modality would destroy *Propionibacterium acnes*, sebaceous glands, or both, and thus, improve acne. The investigators measured pre- and posttreatment sebum excretion rate and autofluorescence from follicular bacteria and histologic changes and protoporphyrin synthesis in pilosebaceous units. ALA was incubated for 3 hours and ALA-induced PpIX was activated with broadband light (550–700 nm) at 150 J/cm^2. One to four treatments were given.

The results showed that ALA-PDT suppressed sebum excretion and bacterial porphyrin fluorescence, caused acute damage to and reduced the size of sebaceous glands, and cleared inflammatory acne vulgaris for 10 to 20 weeks without scarring. Adverse effects included temporary hyperpigmentation, superficial exfoliation, and crusting. A greater amount of ALA-induced PpIX was found in sebaceous glands than in surrounding tissues.

The studies of Divaris and colleagues [43] and Hongcharu and colleagues [45] laid the foundation for the ALA-PDT for acne and SH. Subsequent investigations focused on refining the treatment parameters to improve efficacy and reduce adverse effects.

The study results

Five studies of the use of ALA-PDT for the treatment of SH have been published at the time of this writing (Table 1). The first successful use of ALA-PDT for the treatment of SH was reported by Horio and colleagues [20]. In this study, a 61-year-old Japanese patient with a 10-year history of multiple facial SH lesions (1.5–4.0 mm diameter) sought a nonsurgical treatment with a positive cosmetic result. The ALA-PDT parameters and results are shown in Table 1. Although large papules did not clear completely with three treatment sessions, they became smaller and the initially small papules were nearly eliminated. The encouraging results were maintained for 12 months after treatment. Fluorescence microscopy of a frozen section of one lesion revealed intense red fluorescence in the hyperplastic sebaceous gland, which indicated that topical ALA had penetrated the target tissue adequately. Although burning, edema, erythema, scaling, and pigmentary changes were noted, the treatment was tolerated well.

In a 10-patient study, Alster and Tanzi [52] limited ALA incubation time to 1 hour and used a 595-nm PDL device to activate ALA-induced PpIX. The investigators included two sets of matched SH lesions as controls; one set was not

Table 1
Studies on the use of aminolevulinic acid photodynamic therapy for sebaceous skin

Reference	ALA incubation time (h)	No. of treatments	Light source	Results	Follow-up (mo)
Horio et al [20]	4 (under occlusion)	3	Halogen, >620 nm	Small and large lesions decreased in size and reduced sizes persisted for 12 mo; temporary erythema, edema, hyperpigmentation.	12
Alster et al [52]	1	1, 2	PDL (595 nm)	7 of 10 patients cleared with 1 treatment, 3 patients cleared after 2 treatments; transient erythema, edema, focal crusting.	3
Goldman [54]	0.25	2–4	IPL or blue	Acne and SH lesions cleared after 2–4 treatments.	—
Richey et al [53]	0.75–1	3–6	Blue	70% lesion clearance after 6 mo; 10%–20% recurrence 3–4 mo after final treatment; temporary erythema, edema, hyperpigmentation.	6
Gold et al [55]	0.5–1	4	Blue, IPL	55% reduction in lesions with blue light, 53% with IPL; temporary mild erythema and blisters.	1, 3

Abbreviation: IPL, intense pulsed light.

Adapted from Nestor MS, Gold MH, Kauvar AN, et al. The use of photodynamic therapy in dermatology: results of a consensus conference. J Drugs Dermatol 2006;5(2):148; with permission.

treated and the other set was treated with PDL alone. Patients had at least three large facial lesions (3.0–8.0 mm diameter). PDL treatment parameters were 7.0 J/cm^2 fluence, 6-millisecond pulse duration, and 7-mm spot size. Pulses were double stacked. Each patient received a single treatment and a second treatment 6 weeks later. Improvements were graded on a 0 to 4 scale (0 = <25% of lesion remaining; 4 = >75% of lesion remaining).

Lesions of seven patients (20 lesions) that were treated with ALA-PDT cleared with the initial treatment; lesions of the remaining patients cleared after the second treatment. Mean improvements after a single treatment were 0.3 for lesions treated with ALA-PDT, 1.8 for lesions treated with PDL alone, and 4.0 for untreated lesions. The superior results of ALA-PDT over PDL alone were attributed to the PpIX that formed in the sebaceous glands after ALA pretreatment. Mild stinging was noted only during

laser treatment and no patient required posttreatment pain medication. Focal edema and crusting (which resolved in 2–5 days) were reported in papules in 70% of patients who were treated with ALA-PDT.

Alster and Tanzi [52] obtained complete clearance of most lesions with ALA-PDT, which were larger than those treated by Horio and colleagues. Alster and Tanzi also achieved these results (in most patients) with a single treatment, compared with three treatments by Horio and colleagues [20]. Schonermark and colleagues [22] also required three treatments to clear a single lesion with 585-nm PDL irradiation alone with comparable fluences. Alster and Tanzi reported no hyperpigmentation, whereas Horio and colleagues observed temporary pigmentary changes. The results of Alster and Tanzi suggest that (1) short-contact ALA (1 hour) may provide sufficient penetration of ALA, (2) 595-nm PDL activation may be superior to longer wavelength, broadband activation, and (3) the use of ALA may reduce the number of treatments that is required to clear SH lesions by PDL therapy. The study of Alster and Tanzi is limited by its short (3 month) follow-up time.

Goldman [54] shortened ALA contact time to 15 minutes followed by exposure to blue light or intense pulsed light (IPL) for the treatment of acne or SH by ALA-PDT. The entire face is painted with ALA to treat acne and sebaceous glands that may become acne lesions. Results were considered encouraging because acne and SH lesions cleared after two to four treatments.

Richey and Hopson [53] treated 10 patients (10–50 facial SH lesions, 1–3 mm) with ALA-PDT and 410-nm blue light activation. Patients received three to six weekly treatments and were followed for 6 months. Responses were complete if treated lesions were not visible, and partial if the size of a treated lesion was reduced by 50%. Lesions whose sizes were reduced by less than 50% were considered nonresponders.

Lesions of all patients responded at least partially to ALA-PDT. Lesions became smaller and flattened with each session. On average, 70% of treated lesions cleared completely. Lesions in some patients started to improve after the second or third treatment and continued to improve for up to six treatments. Small papules became smaller or disappeared.

As in the study of Horio and colleagues [20], edema and erythema appeared in treated areas within 1 hour of treatment, reached a maximum at 24 hours, and abated with peeling during the next 4 days. Burning after light exposure was noted in several patients and a blister formed in one patient. Posttreatment skin discoloration and hyperpigmentation in two patients (skin types IV and V) were resolved with hydroquinone within 10 to 21 days. Healing was complete 4 to 7 days after treatment in all patients. Ten to 20% of treated lesions returned 3 to 4 months after the final treatment.

In Richey and Hopson's study [53], 10% to 20% of lesions recurred after 3 to 4 months, whereas in the study of Horio and colleagues [20], lesions did not recur for up to 12 months. The higher recurrence rate in the former study may be due to the shorter ALA contact time, which limited the amount of ALA that penetrated the skin for conversion to PpIX. Horio and colleagues activated ALA-induced PpIX at wavelengths exceeding 620 nm, where absorption of light is much less than at the 410 nm peak that

was used in the author and colleagues' study. Penetration at more than 620 nm is deeper than at 410 nm, however [56].

In the study of Alster and Tanzi [52], a single treatment completely cleared large SH lesions in 70% of patients, possibly because the longer-wavelength laser energy had penetrated deeper into the lesions.

In a 12-patient study, Gold and Goldman [40] evaluated SH lesion counts before and after short-contact ALA-PDT with blue light or IPL activation. Lesion counts were reduced by 55% with blue light activation and by 53% with IPL activation 12 weeks after the final of four monthly treatments. No lesions recurred during the treatment follow-up times. Mild posttreatment erythema persisted for 2 days in two patients, and one blister in a third patient resolved within several days.

The efficacies of blue light and IPL activation are difficult to compare with efficacies in earlier studies because the results are expressed differently and the lesion sizes were not reported in Gold and Goldman's study [40]. Their results, however, suggest that blue light and IPL offer additional options for activation in ALA-PDT for SH.

Consensus recommendation

The consensus recommendations for the treatment of SH by ALA-PDT are to incubate ALA for at least 1 hour (longer if necessary on second or third treatment sessions) before light treatment, and to activate ALA-induced PpIX with (in order of preference) PDL (multiple stacked pulses), blue/IPL, yellow, and red light. Double or triple pulsing on the lesion is recommended when blue light or yellow light is used. One or two treatment sessions that are spaced 2 to 5 weeks apart also are recommended [38].

Summary

ALA-PDT is a safe and effective modality for the treatment of SH lesions of all sizes. One hour seems to be sufficient ALA incubation time and ALA-induced PpIX may be activated with PDL, blue light, or IPL. Complete clearance may be achieved with one to six treatments, but long-term recurrence rates are not established. Additional studies with more patients and other light sources are needed to optimize treatment parameters.

References

[1] Habif TP. Clinical dermatology: a color guide to diagnosis and therapy. 4th edition. New York: Mosby; 2004.

[2] Hogan D, Jones RW, Mason SH. Sebaceous hyperplasia. Available at: http://www.emedicine.com/derm/topic395.htm. Accessed April 14, 2006.

[3] Montagna W. An introduction to sebaceous glands. J Invest Dermatol 1974;62(3):120–3.

[4] Braun-Falco O, Thianprasit M. On circumscribed senile sebaceous gland hyperplasia. Arch Klin Exp Dermatol 1965;221:207–31.

[5] Plewig G, Kligman AM. Proliferative activity of the sebaceous glands of the aged. J Invest Dermatol 1978;70(6):314–7.

[6] Luderschmidt C, Plewig G. Circumscribed sebaceous gland hyperplasia: autoradiographic and histoplanimetric studies. J Invest Dermatol 1978;70(4):207–9.

[7] Bencini PL, Montagnino G, Sala F, et al. Cutaneous lesions in 67 cyclosporin-treated renal transplant recipients. Dermatologica 1986;172(1):24–30.

[8] Walther T, Hohenleutner U, Landthaler M. Sebaceous gland hyperplasia as a side effect of cyclosporin A: treatment with the CO_2 laser. Dtsch Med Wochenschr 1998;123(25–26):798–800.

[9] Grimalt R, Ferrando J, Mascaro JM. Premature familial sebaceous hyperplasia: successful response to oral isotretinoin in three patients. J Am Acad Dermatol 1997;37(6):996–8.

[10] Lynch HT, Fusaro RM, Roberts L, et al. Muir-Torre syndrome in several members of a family with a variant of the Cancer Family Syndrome. Br J Dermatol 1985;113(3):295–301.

[11] Schwartz RA, Torre DP. The Muir-Torre syndrome: a 25-year retrospect. J Am Acad Dermatol 1995;33(1):90–104.

[12] Matsui Y, Nishii Y, Maeda M, et al. [Pachydermoperiostosis–report of a case and review of 121 Japanese cases.] Nippon Hifuka Gakkai Zasshi 1991;101(4):461–7 [in Japanese].

[13] Jansen T, Brandl G, Bandmann M, et al. Pachydermoperiostosis. Hautarzt 1995;46(6):429–35.

[14] Orge C, Bonsmann G, Hamm H. [Multiple sebaceous gland hyperplasias in X chromosome hypohidrotic ectodermal dysplasia.] Hautarzt 1991;42(10):645–7 [in German].

[15] Dupre A, Bonafe JL, Lamon R. Functional familial sebaceous hyperplasia of the face. Reverse of the Cunliffe acne-free naevus? Its inclusion among naevoid sebaceous receptor diseases. Clin Exp Dermatol 1980;5(2):203–7.

[16] De Villez RL, Roberts LC. Premature sebaceous gland hyperplasia. J Am Acad Dermatol 1982;6(5):933–5.

[17] Czarnecki DB, Dorevitch AP. Giant senile sebaceous hyperplasia. Arch Dermatol 1986;122(10):1101.

[18] Uchiyama N, Yamaji K, Shindo Y. Giant solitary sebaceous gland hyperplasia on the frontal region. Dermatologica 1990;181(1):60–1.

[19] Kato N, Yasuoka A. "Giant" senile sebaceous hyperplasia. J Dermatol 1992;19(4):238–41.

[20] Horio T, Horio O, Miyauchi-Hashimoto H, et al. Photodynamic therapy of sebaceous hyperplasia with topical 5-aminolaevulinic acid and slide projector. Br J Dermatol 2003;148:1274–6.

[21] Liu HN, Perry HO. Identifying a common–and benign–geriatric skin lesion. Geriatrics 1986;41(7):71–3 76.

[22] Schonermark MP, Schmidt C, Raulin C. Treatment of sebaceous gland hyperplasia with the pulsed dye laser. Lasers Surg Med 1997;21:313–6.

[23] Aghassi D, Gonzalez E, Anderson RR, et al. Elucidating the pulsed-dye laser treatment of sebaceous hyperplasia in vivo with real-time confocal scanning laser microscopy. J Am Acad Dermatol 2000;43:49–53.

[24] Chanoki M, Izutani K, Maeda T. [Senile sebaceous hyperplasia induced by corticosteroid therapy.] Hifuka No Rinsho 1985;39:897–902 [in Japanese].

[25] Terui T, Takahashi M. [Sebaceous hyperplasia observed in hemodialzyed patient.] Hifuka No Rinsho 1986;28:193–6 [in Japanese].

[26] Stegman SJ. Benign cutaneous tumors and cysts: the importance of biopsy for proper treatment. Postgrad Med 1982;72(4):211–5, 218–21, 224–27.

[27] Blanchet-Bardon C, Servant JM, Le Tuan B, et al. Acquired sebaceous hyperplasia of cutis verticis gyrata type sensitive to 13-cis-retinoid. Ann Dermatol Venereol 1982;109(9):749–50.

[28] Grekin RC, Ellis CN. Isotretinoin for the treatment of sebaceous hyperplasia. Cutis 1984;34(1):90–2.

[29] Burton CS, Sawchuk WS. Premature sebaceous gland hyperplasia: successful treatment with isotretinoin. J Am Acad Dermatol 1985;12(1 Pt 2):182–4.

[30] Wheeland RG, Wiley MD. Q-tip cryosurgery for the treatment of senile sebaceous hyperplasia. J Dermatol Surg Oncol 1987;13(7):729–30.

[31] Rosian R, Goslen JB, Brodell RT. The treatment of benign sebaceous hyperplasia with the topical application of bichloracetic acid. J Dermatol Surg Oncol 1991;17(11):876–9.

[32] Bader RS, Scarborough DA. Surgical pearl: intralesional electrodesiccation of sebaceous hyperplasia. J Am Acad Dermatol 2000;42(1 Pt 1):127–8.

[33] Landthaler M, Haina D, Waidelich W, et al. A three-year experience with the argon laser in dermatotherapy. J Dermatol Surg Oncol 1984;10(6):456–61.

[34] Marsili M, Cockerell CJ, Lyde CB. Hemangioma-associated rhinophyma. Report of a case with successful treatment using carbon dioxide laser surgery. J Dermatol Surg Oncol 1993;19(3):206–12.

[35] Gonzalez S, White WM, Rajadhyaksha M, et al. Confocal imaging of sebaceous gland hyperplasia in vivo to assess efficacy and mechanism of pulsed

dye laser treatment. Lasers Surg Med 1999;25(1): 8–12.

[36] No D, McClaren M, Chotzen V, et al. Sebaceous hyperplasia treated with a 1450-nm diode laser. Dermatol Surg 2004;30(3):382–4.

[37] Schonermark MP, Raulin C. Treatment of xanthelasma palpebrarum with the pulsed dye laser. Lasers Surg Med 1996;19(3):336–9.

[38] Nestor MS, Gold MH, Kauvar AN, et al. The use of photodynamic therapy in dermatology: results of a consensus conference. J Drugs Dermatol 2006; 5(2):140–54.

[39] Taub AF. Photodynamic therapy in dermatology: history and horizons. J Drugs Dermatol 2004; 3(Suppl 1):8–25.

[40] Gold MH, Goldman MP. 5-aminolevulinic acid photodynamic therapy: where we have been and where we are going. Dermatol Surg 2004;30: 1077–83.

[41] Kennedy JC, Pottier RH, Pross DC. Photodynamic therapy with endogenous protoporphyrin IX: basic principles and present clinical experience. J Photochem Photobiol B 1990;6:143–8.

[42] Kennedy JC, Pottier RH. Endogenous protoporphyrin IX, a clinically useful photosensitizer for photodynamic therapy. J Photochem Photobiol B 1992; 14:275–92.

[43] Divaris DX, Kennedy JC, Pottier RH. Phototoxic damage to sebaceous glands and hair follicles of mice after systemic administration of 5-aminolevulinic acid correlates with localized protoporphyrin IX fluorescence. Am J Pathol 1990;136(4):891–7.

[44] Cunliffe WJ, Goulden V. Phototherapy and acne vulgaris. Br J Dermatol 2000;142:855–6.

[45] Hongcharu W, Taylor CR, Chang Y, et al. Topical ALA-photodynamic therapy for the treatment of acne vulgaris. J Invest Dermatol 2000;115(2):183–92.

[46] Itoh Y, Ninomiya Y, Tajima S, et al. Photodynamic therapy for acne vulgaris with topical 5-aminolevulinic acid. Arch Dermatol 2000;136:1093–5.

[47] Itoh Y, Ninomiya Y, Tajima S, et al. Photodynamic therapy of acne vulgaris with topical delta-aminolevulinic acid and incoherent light in Japanese patients. Br J Dermatol 2001;144:575–9.

[48] Goldman MP, Boyce SM. A single-center study of aminolevulinic acid and 417 NM photodynamic therapy in the treatment of moderate to severe acne vulgaris. J Drugs Dermatol 2003; 2(4):393–6.

[49] Gold MH. The utilization of ALA PDT and a new photoclearing device for the treatment of severe inflammatory acne vulgaris—results of an initial clinical trial. J Lasers Surg Med 2003; 15(Suppl):46.

[50] Taub A. Photodynamic therapy for the treatment of acne: a pilot study. J Drugs Dermatol 2004; 3(Suppl 6):10–4.

[51] Alexiades-Armenakas M. Long-pulsed dye laser-mediated photodynamic therapy combined with topical therapy for mild to severe comedonal, inflammatory, or cystic acne. J Drugs Dermatol 2006;5(1):45–55.

[52] Alster TS, Tanzi EL. Photodynamic therapy with topical aminolevulinic acid and pulsed dye laser irradiation for sebaceous hyperplasia. J Drugs Dermatol 2003;2:501–4.

[53] Richey DF, Hopson B. Treatment of sebaceous hyperplasia by photodynamic therapy. Cosmetic Dermatol 2004;17:525–9.

[54] Goldman MP. Using 5-aminolevulinic acid to treat acne and sebaceous hyperplasia. Cosmetic Dermatol 2003;16:57–8.

[55] Gold MH, Bradshaw VL, Boring MM, et al. Treatment of sebaceous gland hyperplasia by photodynamic therapy with 5-aminolevulinic acid and a blue light source or intense pulsed light source. J Drugs Dermatol 2004;3(6 Suppl):6–9.

[56] Wilson BC, Patterson MS. The physics of photodynamic therapy. Phys Med Biol 1986;31: 327–60.

Aminolevulinic Acid Photodynamic Therapy for Hidradenitis Suppurativa

Michael H. Gold, MD[a,b,*]

[a]Gold Skin Care Center, Tennessee Clinical Research Center, 2000 Richard Jones Road,
Suite 220, Nashville, TN 37215, USA
[b]Vanderbilt University Medical School, Vanderbilt University Nursing School,
Nashville, TN 37215, USA

Hidradenitis suppurativa (HS) is a chronic, often suppurativa dermatologic disorder that principally affects apocrine gland–bearing skin. HS is a disease that has been misdiagnosed often, is not studied adequately by clinical researchers, and often is not treated appropriately by clinicians.

Human sweat glands were described first by Purkinje in 1833 [1]. HS was described first in the medical literature by Velpeau in 1833 [2]. It was several years later, in 1845, that Robin [3] described the structure, function, and location of human apocrine glands. HS was related to apocrine gland structure and function by Verneuil in 1854 [4], when he described "hydrosadenite phlegmoneuse" as an apocrine gland disorder, later to be known simply as HS. Little clinical research ensued for some time. It was not until 1955 that Shelley and Cahn [5] reported that the cause of HS includes keratinous plugging, dilatation, and severe inflammation of the apocrine duct. Published reports in the 1990s showed that HS is an acne vulgaris-like disorder, with predominant follicular occlusion; the apocrine glands play a role mainly in the associated perifollicular inflammatory response [6–9].

The exact cause and prevalence of HS are unknown, because many patients who suffer from HS do not present to physicians for treatment and because physicians often misdiagnose the disease. Prevalence rates for HS are estimated to be from 1 in 100 to 1 in 600 individuals, based on several studies [10–12]. This translates into approximately 100,000 patients who have HS in the United Kingdom and more than 400,000 patients in the United States. Further estimates state that 1% of the population is at risk for the development of HS (ie, >2 million United States adults may suffer from HS).

HS seems to have a genetic predisposition, and clinical studies showed that between 13% and 38% of patients report a family history of HS. An autosomal dominant and an autosomal recessive type of inheritance pattern have been described. HS is more predominant in women, with a female/male predominance reported to be as high as 4:1. Female patients who have HS note increased disease symptoms associated with menses. Dermatologic Life Quality Index studies demonstrated that patients who have HS have a higher impairment rating than do those who have other skin disorders studied, including acne vulgaris, eczema, or psoriasis [12–15].

HS has been described most commonly as a primary skin condition. On occasion, HS has been associated with other skin disorders (Box 1).

The clinical presentation of HS has been described well. Inflammatory cystic lesions appear in the predominant apocrine gland–bearing skin, especially the skin of the axillae and the inguinal region. Other apocrine gland areas of the skin that can show signs and symptoms of HS include

Dr. Gold is a consultant for Dusa Pharmaceuticals, speaks on their behalf, receives honoraria, and performs research on their behalf. Dr. Gold also is a consultant for numerous pharmaceutical and device companies and performs research on their behalf.

* Gold Skin Care Center, Tennessee Clinical Research Center, 2000 Richard Jones Road, Suite 220, Nashville, TN 37215.

E-mail address: goldskin@goldskincare.com

Box 1. Diseases with an association with HS

Crohn's disease
Irritable bowel syndrome
Down's syndrome
Arthritis
Graves disease
Hashimoto thyroiditis
Sjögren's syndrome
Hyperandrogenism
Herpes simplex
Acanthosis nigricans

inframammary areas, perineal areas, buttocks, scrotum, mons pubis, and abdominal folds [16].

The typical lesion of HS is described as a painful inflammatory papule, nodule, or abscess. These lesions usually remain tender for several days to approximately 1 week. Lesions may be found in different stages at different times on the same individual, and, on occasion, chronic lesions never resolve. This results in the formation of abscesses that can lead to the development of intradermal or subcutaneous epithelial-lined sinus tracts, which continue to be a source of intense inflammatory activity. A recent clinical trial showed, that on average, individuals who suffer from HS have 4.8 inflammatory lesions each month, and that disease activity lasted upwards of 20 years in this cohort of individuals [17].

Typically, three phases of HS are described [12,18]:

- Primary stage: boils appear in separate places and where nodular noninflamed precursor lesions appear.
- Secondary stage: sinus tracts appear with scarring linking individual lesions.
- Tertiary stage: coalescing, scarring, and sinus tracts predominate although inflammation and chronic discharge also appear (Figs. 1 and 2).

The histologic findings are shown in Figs. 3 and 4 [18]. Several factors aggravate HS, including stress, heat, sweating, and friction. More than 50% of women report a flare of the disease with their menstrual cycle. Smoking may have some role in triggering flares of HS; more than 70% of sufferers of HS smoke, a higher rate than would be expected in the general population [19,20].

The treatment of HS remains difficult and frustrating for the patient and for the physician. Most physicians should approach the therapy of HS on two fronts: treating acute disease flare-ups and considering the long-term management of this chronic disease. It is beyond the scope of this article to review all of the clinical trials that are related to the therapy of HS thoroughly. The treatment of acute disease flare-ups varies from medical to surgical intervention. Medical management in the dermatology arena includes systemic and topical antibiotics and systemic and intralesional corticosteroids. Hormonal intervention also has been used, with mixed results. The efficacies of these

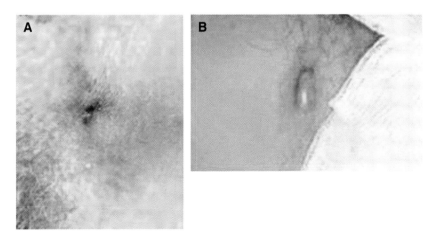

Fig. 1. Clinical examples of stage 1 (*A*) and 2 (*B*) HS. (*From* Sartorius K, Lapins J, Emtestam L. Suggestions for uniform outcome variables when reporting treatment effects in hidradenitis suppurativa. Br J Dermatol 2003;149(1):211–3; with permission.)

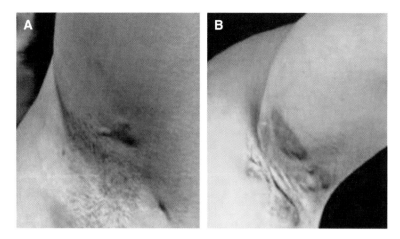

Fig. 2. Clinical examples of stage 3 HS (*A,B*). (*From* Sartorius K, Lapins J, Emtestam L. Suggestions for uniform outcome variables when reporting treatment effects in hidradenitis suppurativa. Br J Dermatol 2003;149(1):211–3; with permission.)

medical therapies are disputed by many authorities, although most would argue that their use is still the first line of therapy. Systemic isotretinoin also has been used with mixed results in patients who have HS. Newer medical therapies include the use of the psoriasis biologic medications (eg, infliximab, etanercept, efalizumab). Clinical studies are ongoing to determine if these anti–tumor necrosis factor medications play a role in suppressing the disease process [16].

Many investigators suggest surgical modalities as the major mainstay in the management of HS. Incision and drainage, probably the most common of the HS treatment modalities performed, may make the entire area more inflamed, which worsens the overall disease process. Excision of small areas of disease activity may be performed; however, most surgeons would argue that wide, radical surgical excision may be the only way to control the disease. Most dermatologists would argue that they all have seen cases in which wide surgical excision did not halt the disease progression and might make further therapies more difficult. Lasers, such as the CO_2 laser, also have been used, again with mixed results [16].

The rest of this article deals with the use of photodynamic therapy (PDT) in the treatment of HS. PDT uses a photosensitizer, molecular oxygen, and light to destroy certain cells in the body selectively. Dermatologic uses of PDT rely on

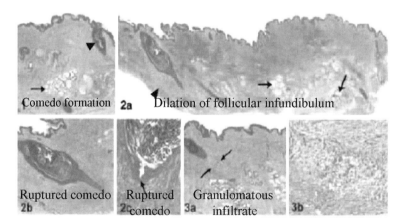

Fig. 3. Histologic findings. (*From* Sellheyer K, Krahl D. "Hidradenitis suppurativa" is acne inversa! An appeal to (finally) abandon a misnomer. Int J Dermatol 2005;44:535–40; with permission.)

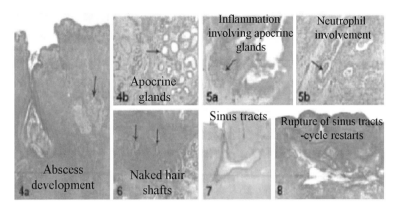

Fig. 4. Histologic findings. (*From* Sellheyer K, Krahl D. "Hidradenitis suppurativa" is acne inversa! An appeal to (finally) abandon a misnomer. Int J Dermatol 2005;44:535–40; with permission.)

20% 5-aminolevulinic acid (ALA). The two available photosensitizers are Levulan Kerastick (Dusa Pharmaceuticals, Wilmington, Massachusetts) and Metvix (PhotoCure ASA, Oslo, Norway). At the time of this writing, only Levulan Kerastick is available in the United States. The FDA approval for Levulan is for the treatment of non-hyperkeratotic actinic keratoses (AKs) of the face and scalp using a blue light source after a drug incubation time of 14 to 18 hours. The European Union clearance for Metvix is for nonhyperkeratotic AKs of the face and scalp, as well as superficial basal cell carcinomas that are unsuitable for conventional therapy. It also is cleared in the United States for the treatment of AKs, although it is not available at this time. The recommended use of this methyl ester of ALA is to apply the cream to the affected area, occlude for 3 hours, and to use a red light source at 630 nm. The use of any of these photosensitizers in the treatment of HS is considered an off-label use of the product; it is imperative for the physician to explain this to all patients who receive this type of therapy for the treatment of HS [20].

The clinical uses of Levulan Kerastick and Metvix have been reviewed in numerous drafts (also see elsewhere in this issue). They are not covered in detail here. In the United States, Levulan is used most commonly as a short-contact, full-face contact therapy, especially for the treatment of photorejuvenation with associated AKs, acne vulgaris, and sebaceous gland hyperplasia. A variety of lasers and light sources is used commonly with Levulan, based on the absorption characteristics to light of protoporphyrin IX (PpIX (Fig. 5). Metvix, used with the 3-hour drug incubation under occlusion in Europe, is used most commonly to treat superficial nonmelanoma skin cancers, AKs, and Bowen's disease with a red light source at 630 nm [21].

With this background, and with the understanding that ALA penetrates into sebaceous glands, the author and his colleagues [16] reported on the use of Levulan in the treatment of HS in 2004. Four patients who had recalcitrant HS were identified and treated with short-contact ALA and then exposed to a blue light source. The drug incubation time was between 15 and 30 minutes, and exposure to the blue light lasted for an average of 18 minutes. Each patient received three or four treatments at 1- to 2-week intervals and was followed over time. Clearance was noted in 75% to 100% of the patients at the 3-month follow-up period. Clinical examples are shown in Figs. 6 and 7.

Because HS predominantly is an apocrine disorder, and not a sebaceous gland problem, it is difficult to explain how ALA-PDT works in recalcitrant HS. There is selective accumulation of PpIX in the hair follicle epithelium associated with the sebaceous glands near the disease pathology; with proper light exposure, as seen in patients who have inflammatory acne vulgaris, a PDT reaction can occur. As well, a potent anti-inflammatory response may play a major role in the resolution of these lesions. As a follow-up to the cases already presented, three of the four patients have remained disease free for more than 3 years now. The fourth patient requires maintenance therapy approximately every 6 months because his disease process has waxed and waned; each time it responds positively to the ALA-PDT therapy.

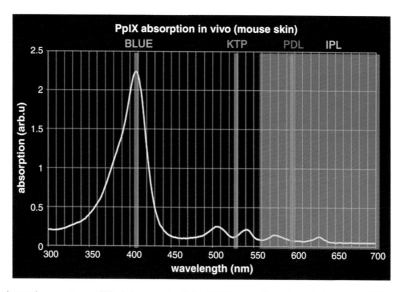

Fig. 5. PpIX absorption spectrum. IPL, intense pulse light; KTP, potassium titanyl phosphate; PDL, pulse dye laser.

Another report in the literature, this time using the methyl ester cream, did not show results that were as positive as those of the United States experience. In 2005, Strauss and colleagues [22] reported their findings with four patients who had recalcitrant HS. They used Metvix with a drug incubation of 4 hours under occlusion. Before each light treatment, local anesthesia was given to each site. A Ceramoptic diode laser (633 nm) was used in three patients and a broadband light source (570–640 nm) was used in one patient. Each patient was scheduled to receive three weekly treatments with an 8-week follow-up period. One of the patients received three treatments and one received two treatments; of these two patients, one improved and one worsened. One of the other patients did not complete the therapy because of adverse events (severe burning and stinging), and one patient had two treatments but did not continue because of worsening of the disease process. The investigators concluded that PDT was not useful in cases of HS.

Many issues can be raised in the study that was performed by Strauss and colleagues [22], including the use of the methyl ester under occlusion for 4 hours and then exposure to the light source. The explanation that apocrine gland activity is deep in the dermal tissue and that long drug incubation is required may or may not be relevant if we are relying on a resultant potent anti-inflammatory response to help resolve disease activity. This long drug incubation time, along with local anesthesia and red light therapy, are painful and can cause significant PDT effects, or downtime, as was described previously [21]. The short-contact blue light therapy resulted in a presumed

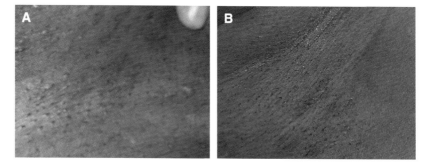

Fig. 6. Clinical examples of recalcitrant HS (A, B).

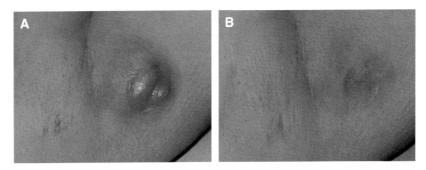

Fig. 7. Clinical examples of recalcitrant HS (*A, B*).

anti-inflammatory response and resolution of HS lesions, all without significant discomfort and no patient downtime.

Larger and more controlled clinical trials are warranted for the treatment of HS with ALA-PDT. This can be such a disabling disorder and patients are looking for new therapies that can alleviate their symptoms, in the short and long term. ALA-PDT may be one of those answers. We owe it to our patients to study this disease further and to develop newer therapies for these individuals. The author encourages clinicians to discuss this issue with pharmaceutical companies that are involved in ALA-PDT treatments to help fund these important clinical trials, again in the hope of providing relief, temporary or long-term, for these patients.

References

[1] Gordon SW. Hidradenitis suppurativa: a closer look. J Natl Med Assoc 1978;70:339–43.

[2] Velpeau A. Dictionnaire de médecine, un répertoire général des sciences médicales sous la rapport théorique et practique, vol. 2. 2nd edition. Paris: Bechet Jeune; 1833. p. 91–109 [in French].

[3] Robin C. Note sur une espece particuliere de glandes de la peau de l'homme. Troisieme serie Zoologie Ann Sci Nat Paris 1845;4:380 [in French].

[4] Verneuil A. De l'hidrosadenite phlegmoneuse et des abces sudoripares. Arch Gen Med 1854;2:537–57 [in French].

[5] Shelley WB, Cahn MM. The pathogenesis of hidradenitis suppurativa. Arch Dermatol 1955;72: 562–5.

[6] Yu CC, Cook MG. Hidradenitis suppurativa: a disease of follicular epithelium, rather than apocrine glands. Br J Dermatol 1990;122(6):763–9.

[7] Attanoos RL, Appleton MA, Douglas-Jones AG. The pathogenesis of hidradenitis suppurativa: a closer look at apocrine and apoecrine glands. Br J Dermatol 1995;133(2):254–8.

[8] Layton AM, Pace D, Cunliffe WJ, et al. A perspective histological study of acute hidradenitis suppurativa. Br J Dermatol 1995;131(S44):38–9.

[9] Jemec GB, Hansen U. Histology of hidradenitis suppurativa. J Am Acad Dermatol 1996;34(6): 994–9.

[10] Harrison BJ, Mudge M, Hughes LE. The prevalence of hidradenitis suppurativa in South Wales. In: Marks R, Plewig G, editors. Acne and related disorders. London: Martin Dunitz; 1991. p. 365–6.

[11] Fitzsimmons JS, Guilbert PR. A family study of hidradenitis suppurativa. J Med Genet 1985;22(5): 367–73.

[12] Sartorius K, Lapins J, Emtestam L. Suggestions for uniform outcome variables when reporting treatment effects in hidradenitis suppurativa. Br J Dermatol 2003;149(1):211–3.

[13] Von der Werth JM, Williams HC, Raeburn JA. The clinical genetics of hidradenitis suppurativa revisited. Br J Dermatol 2000;142:947–57.

[14] Galen WK, Cohen I, Roger M, et al. Bacterial infections. In: Schachner LA, Hansen RC, editors. Pediatric dermatology. 2nd edition. New York: Churchill Livingstone; 1996. p. 1206–7.

[15] Von der Werth JM, Jemec GB. Morbidity in patients with hidradenitis suppurativa. Br J Dermatol 2001; 144(4):809–13.

[16] Gold MH, Bridges TM, Bradshaw VL, et al. ALA-PDT and blue light therapy for hidradenitis suppurativa. J Drugs Dermatol 2004;3(s):32–9.

[17] Von der Werth JM, Williams HC. The natural history of hidradenitis suppurativa. J Eur Acad Dermatol Venereol 2000;14(5):389–92.

[18] Selheyer K, Krahl D. "Hidradenitis suppurativa" is acne inversa! Int J Dermatol 2005;44(7):535–40.

[19] Wiltz O, Schoetz DJ Jr, Murray JJ, et al. Perianal hidradenitis suppurativa. The Lahey Clinic experience. Dis Colon Rectum 1990;33(9):731–4.

[20] Breitkopf C, Bockhurt J, Lippold A, et al. Pyoderma fistulans sinifica (akne inversa) und eauchgewohnheiten. Z Haut 1995;70:332–4.

[21] Gold MH, Goldman MP. 5-Aminolevulinic acid photodynamic therapy: where we have been and where we are going. Dermatol Surg 2004;30: 1077–84.

[22] Strauss RM, Pollock B, Stables GI, et al. Photodynamic therapy using aminolaevulinic acid does not lead to improvement in hidradenitis suppurativa. Br J Dermatol 2005;152:803–4.

ELSEVIER
SAUNDERS

Dermatol Clin 25 (2007) 75–80

DERMATOLOGIC
CLINICS

Treatment of Verrucae Vulgaris and Molluscum Contagiosum with Photodynamic Therapy

Michael H. Gold, MD[a,b,*], Ali Moiin, MD[c]

[a]Gold Skin Care Center, Tennessee Clinical Research Center,
2000 Richard Jones Road, Suite 220, Nashville, TN 37215, USA
[b]Vanderbilt University Medical School, Vanderbilt University Nursing School, Nashville, TN 37215, USA
[c]Department of Dermatology, Wayne State University School of Medicine,
4717 Saint Antoine Street, Detroit, MI 48201, USA

Photodynamic therapy (PDT) with 20% 5-aminolevulinc acid (ALA) has shown to be effective for a variety of dermatologic skin concerns. These include the treatment of actinic keratoses with or without photorejuvenation, acne vulgaris and related entities, and nonmelanoma skin cancers. These have been outlined and reviewed in elsewhere in this issue.

The Food and Drug Administration approval for ALA in the United States is for the treatment of nonhyperkeratotic actinic keratoses of the face and scalp, using a blue light source and a drug incubation time of 14 to 18 hours [1]. All other uses are considered off-label at the time of this writing.

This article reviews the published data on the use of ALA-PDT in the treatment of recalcitrant verrucae vulgaris and recalcitrant molluscum contagiosum. Clinical papers in the medical literature and personal experience of both of the authors support the use in ALA-PDT in appropriate individuals.

Verrucae are double-stranded DNA viral entities, caused by the human papilloma virus, a member of the Papovaviridae family. They are very common manifestations in dermatology offices and have been identified in virtually all parts of the body, with many (>70) genotypes being identified. Both skin and mucosal surfaces can be affected by these lesions. Warts are clinically identified as papular or nodular structures that have a horny layer on their surface; they can range from 1 to 2 mm in size to several centimeters and may become confluent leading to the appearance of even larger lesions. Pain and functional abnormalities have been reported as a result of verrucous lesions on the hands and feet. Epidemiologic evidence has shown up to 22% of school-age children develop verrucous lesions and upwards of 50% to 95% of renal transplant patients develop verrucous lesions that may progress toward squamous cell carcinomas [2].

Histologic analyses of verrucous lesions shows hyperplasia of the epidermis, along with acanthosis, papillomatosis, hyperkeratosis with parakeratosis, and thrombosed capillaries in the dermal papillae. Elongated rete ridges curve, in most incidences, to the center of the lesion. Viral replication takes place in differentiated keratinocytes in or above the stratum granulosum. Vacuolated cells, known as "koilocytotic cells," are found in the mid-upper dermis [2].

Treatments of verrucae are often discouraging to both the patient and clinician and numerous manuscripts have summarized therapeutic options for these clinical lesions. Treatment options

Dr. Gold is a consultant for Dusa Pharmaceuticals, speaks on their behalf, receives honoraria, and performs research on their behalf. Dr. Gold is also a consultant for numerous pharmaceutical and device companies and performs research on their behalf.

* Corresponding author. Gold Skin Care Center, Tennessee Clinical Research Center, 2000 Richard Jones Road, Suite 220, Nashville, TN 37215.

  E-mail address: goldskin@goldskincare.com (M.H. Gold).

usually focus on the physical destruction of the lesion (ie, the viral cell) and include cryotherapy [3], curettage, excision, carbon dioxide laser ablation [4], pulsed dye laser therapy [5], liquid nitrogen, electrosurgery, and the application of a variety of topical acid preparations [6,7]. Other modalities reported in the dermatologic literature include the use of infrared coagulation [8], interferon-α, topically applied 5-flurouracil [9], intralesional bleomycin [10], and the use of topically applied dinitrochlorobenzene [11]. Despite these treatment modalities, some warts remain recalcitrant to the therapies.

Molluscum contagiosum are also caused by viruses, these being large DNA pox viruses. They are commonly seen in children and have had resurgence in those afflicted with HIV disease [12–17]. They are clinically described as being discrete skin-colored smooth papules with an umbilicated center. These lesions occur on both the skin and mucous membranes. In children, lesions are reported to occur on all body surfaces; those in HIV-positive individuals are more commonly described on the skin surfaces of the head and neck area. They are also reported to be larger than the typical small papular lesions seen in children and are in general more recalcitrant to therapeutic options [18].

The incidence of molluscum lesions is reported to be as high as 5% in children and up to 5% to 18% in the HIV and immunocompromised population. Histologic examination shows a hypertrophied and hyperplastic epidermis. Above the basal layer there are lobules of enlarged epidermal cells with inclusion bodies, commonly known as "molluscum bodies." The inclusion bodies contain the viral particles [16,18,19–23].

Treatment options for molluscum are numerous, and similar to those described for verrucous lesions. Typical treatment modalities include liquid nitrogen, cantharidin, tretinoin cream, podophyllin 20% to 25%, salicylic acid, tincture of iodine, silver nitrate, trichloroacetic acid, and surgery with curettage with or without electrical desiccation. In HIV-positive individuals, antiretroviral therapy, intralesional interferon-α, and injection of streptococcal antigen OK-432 have been reported to be useful in treating molluscum. Despite these modalities, recalcitrant lesions are often reported [15].

PDT is a therapeutic modality that uses a photosensitizer and light, which in the presence of oxygen and an appropriate light source causes selective cell death. This leads to clearance of the affected lesion. The primary dermatologic uses of PDT have been reported elsewhere in this issue.

PDT has been reported in the treatment of recalcitrant verrucous lesions and molluscum lesions over the past 10 years. These studies are summarized next. In the first pilot series published in 1995, Ammann and coworkers [24] reported their findings using PDT in six patients with refractory verrucae vulgaris of the hands. These patients were all treatment failures and the duration of their verrucous lesions were from 2 to 10 years. They used 20% ALA in an oil-in-water emulsion, which was applied under occlusion for 5 to 6 hours before being illuminated using a slide projector light source for 30 minutes. The patients were followed for up to 2 months after their therapy. The treated areas in all the patients studied showed an acute inflammatory skin reaction. In five of the individuals, there was no change in the verrucae; however, in one patient complete resolution of the verrucae was achieved. The authors noted that in this series, PDT was not a success in the treatment of verrucae, but were encouraged by the one treatment success and suggested further research into the field of study.

In 1997, Smetana and coworkers [25] reported on their experiences with in vivo and in vitro analyses using PDT in both verrucae and molluscum patients. In their verrucous case report, a 15-year kidney transplant patient presented with recalcitrant verrucae on the hands. A 20% ALA cream containing 2% ethylenediaminetetraacetic acid and 2% dimethyl sulfoxide was applied to the affected areas and incubated for a period of 4 hours. Red light was used to activate the photosensitizer, at 120 J/cm². Dramatic improvement was noted at the 1-month follow-up period. No recurrence was noted 2 years later. Their second patient, an HIV-positive individual, presented with molluscum lesions on the face area. Using a similar protocol, the authors achieved similar clearance at the 1-month follow-up period. The authors concluded that ALA-PDT may be a useful modality for recalcitrant verrucae and molluscum, especially with the additives that were added to the ALA preparation.

Stender and coworkers [26], in 2000, published their findings in 232 hand and foot verrucous lesions found in 45 individuals. They randomized 117 lesions to receive ALA-PDT and 115 to receive placebo-PDT. Each lesion was treated with occlusion of the affected area for 4 hours and the lesions were irradiated with a red light source (Waldman PDT 1200, Waldmann-Medizin-Technik,

Villingen-Schwenningen, Germany), with a wavelength range of 590 to 700 nm. The lesions were exposed to 50 J/cm^2 for 23 minutes and 20 seconds, yielding a total dose of 70 J/cm^2. All of the verrucae were treated at baseline, at 1 week, and at 2 weeks, with another treatment regimen of three treatments given 1 month later if clearance was not achieved. Follow-up was at 1 and 2 months following the last treatment. Their results were as follows: at week 14, there was a relative reduction in wart area of 98% in the ALA group versus 52% in the placebo group. At week 18, the relative reduction in the ALA group was 100% versus 71% in the placebo group. Pain was more evident in the ALA-treated group compared with the placebo group. The authors concluded their study supported the use of ALA-PDT in the treatment of recalcitrant verrucae.

Fabbrocini and coworkers [27], in 2001, reported their experience with recalcitrant plantar warts. They evaluated 67 patients using PDT in these recalcitrant lesions. Each lesion was pretreated for 7 days with a topical ointment containing 10% urea and 10% salicylic acid to remove the superficial hyperkeratotic layers commonly seen in these lesions. A gentle curettage was also used before the application of the ALA; the ALA was a 20% cream preparation using Eucerin cream as its base. The ALA was occluded for 5 hours. Sixty-four lesions received the ALA cream, whereas 57 warts received only the Eucerin cream base. The photoactivator used was a tungsten lamp that emitted a spectrum of light from 400 to 700 nm, with a peak at 630 nm. The power incidence was 50 mW/cm^2, at a distance of 10 cm. Patients received one treatment, and if not clear, received two more therapies at 1-week intervals; they were then followed for 22 months. Their results showed that 48 (75%) of 64 warts completely healed compared with 13 (22.8%) out of the 57 lesions in the placebo group. Of interest, 47.9% of the ALA lesions cleared following one treatment, 31.3% required two treatments, and only 20.8% needed three treatments for clearance to occur. The authors concluded that ALA was successful in the treatment of recalcitrant verrucae.

Stender and coworkers [28], in 1999, reported further work on the use of ALA-PDT in the treatment of recalcitrant verrucae of the hands and feet. They evaluated 30 individuals with a total of 250 verrucous lesions and randomized patients to receive one of five treatment protocols: ALA-PDT with white light three times in 10 days; ALA-PDT with white light for one treatment; ALA-PDT with red light for three treatments in 10 days; ALA-PDT with blue light for three treatments in 10 days; and cryotherapy, up to four treatments within a 2-month period. The ALA used was a 20% ALA preparation; each lesion was incubated for 5 hours under occlusion. The areas treated were illuminated with light from slide projectors (halogen lamp) at a distance of 15 cm, with a total dose given of 40 J/cm^2. The treatments were repeated if the lesions were not completely cleared after the first course. The results from the study showed complete clearance of 73% with white light with three treatments, 71% after one white light treatment, 42% after red light therapy, 23% after blue light therapy, and 20% after cryotherapy. Of the areas that cleared, no recurrences were noted after a 12-month follow-up period. The authors concluded that ALA-PDT is a useful modality for the treatment of recalcitrant verrucae of the hands and feet.

Mizuki and coworkers [29], in 2003, reported on the use of ALA-PDT in a 13-year-old Japanese boy who had a 2-year history of multiple "plane" warts of the face, unresponsive to previous therapies. They used a 20% ALA oil-in-water emulsion and a single 500-W metal halide lamp with peaks of 630 and 700 nm. The ALA was incubated for 6 hours under occlusion; illumination was for 20 minutes for energy of 120 J/cm^2. The patient underwent two ALA-PDT sessions. Five months after the final treatment, the areas remained disease free. This suggested ALA-PDT was useful for the treatment of recalcitrant plane warts.

Smucler and Jatsova [30], in 2005, reported on the use of a pulsed dye laser with ALA in the treatment of verrucous lesions. They compared pulsed dye laser alone versus pulsed dye laser plus PDT and PDT and a light-emitting diode light source. They found that all three of their protocols were effective in treating these recalcitrant lesions, but the combination of pulsed dye laser plus PDT resulted in the highest cure rate with the shortest number of treatments. Pulsed dye laser cured 81% of the lesions treated (N = 112), with a mean number of sessions being 3.34. Pulsed dye laser plus PDT cured 100% (N = 86), with a mean number of sessions being 1.95. PDT plus light-emitting diode cured 96% of the lesions (N = 76), with a mean number of sessions being 2.53. The authors strongly suggested this combined modality to become a treatment of choice for viral warts.

Gold [31] reported on the successful use of ALA-PDT in the treatment of recalcitrant molluscum contagiosum in an HIV individual in 2004.

After discussions about similar successes with Orenstein, the group treated an HIV-positive individual with four sessions of ALA-PDT using the original Food and Drug Administration treatment protocol. The ALA used was Levulan Kerastick (Dusa Pharmaceuticals, Wilmington, Massachusetts). Its use has been fully reviewed elsewhere in this issue. The ALA was applied to individual lesions and allowed to incubate for 16 hours before exposure to a blue light source (ClearLight, CureLight, Yokneam, Israel) for 16 minutes and 40 seconds. The therapy was reported painful during the illumination, so cool water and a fan was used to ease this discomfort. There was a significant inflammatory response following each treatment, which required systemic and topical corticosteroids for relief. The treatments were performed at 2-week intervals and a dramatic response was seen after the fourth treatment.

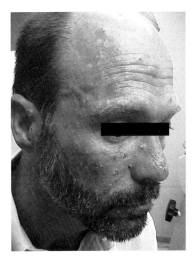

Fig. 1. ALA was applied broadly to the affected areas, incubated from 14 to 24 hours, and treated with the blue light for 16 minutes and 40 seconds. Improvements in their lesion count were realized.

Box 1. **Patient inclusion-exclusion criteria**

Inclusion criteria
- Male and nonpregnant female outpatients, 18 years and older
- Presence of suspected molluscum contagiosum
- Written informed patient consent
- HIV positive

Exclusion criteria
- A history of cutaneous photosensitization, porphyria, hypersensitivity to porphyrins, or photodermatoses
- A known sensitivity to the use of Levulan or any of its vehicle components
- Uncorrected coagulation defects
- Pregnant or lactating patients

Prior therapy washout
- No treatment within 1 month: systemic steroid therapy or topical treatment with any other investigational drug
- No treatment within 2 months: laser resurfacing, chemical peels, topical application of 5-flurorouracil for treatment of molluscum contagiosum virus, systemic treatment with chemotherapeutic agents, psoralens, or immunotherapy

---

Moiin, in preparation of this manuscript, reviewed 40 patients with molluscum lesions treated with Levulan Kerastick and a blue light source, the BluU (Dusa Pharmaceuticals, Wilmington, Massachusetts). Six of the individuals reviewed also had a history of HIV infection, and are the basis of this report. The ALA was applied broadly to the affected areas, incubated from 14 to 24 hours, and treated with the blue light for 16 minutes and 40 seconds. All of the patients studied improved in their lesion count, as shown in Box 1 and demonstrated in Figs. 1–3. In two patients, one treatment produced an improvement

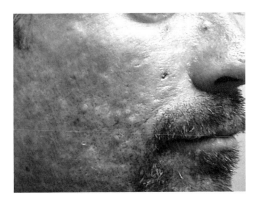

Fig. 2. ALA was applied broadly to the affected areas, incubated from 14 to 24 hours, and treated with the blue light for 16 minutes and 40 seconds. Improvements in their lesion count were realized.

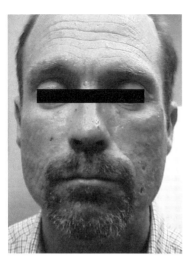

Fig. 3. ALA was applied broadly to the affected areas, incubated from 14 to 24 hours, and treated with the blue light for 16 minutes and 40 seconds. Improvements in their lesion count were realized.

in the lesion count of 60%. Furthermore, patients who received three to five treatments were found to have a 75% to 80% reduction in the number of lesions counted. The therapy did yield a phototoxic reaction that included erythema, edema, vesiculation, hyperpigmentation, hypopigmentation, pain, stinging and burning, and itching (Fig. 4). The only deliberately intense side effect was a burning sensation described by one patient when placed under the blue light source. Only one child did not tolerate the procedure fully because of erythema formation. The conclusion is that PDT is a viable option for treating molluscum

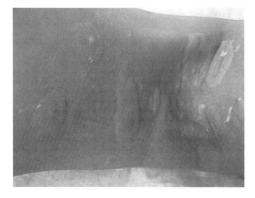

Fig. 4. Patient experienced phototoxic reaction including erythema, edema, vesiculation, hyperpigmentation, hypopigmentation, pain, stinging and burning, and itching.

contagiosum in HIV-positive patients and immunocompromised children. All of the patients expressed preference of ALA-PDT over previous therapies for their molluscum.

The use of ALA-PDT has been shown to be successful for the treatment of recalcitrant verrucae and molluscum contagiosum lesions. Studies have shown that ALA-PDT is a useful modality for these lesions and should be considered when confronted with a patient with either of these viral conditions. Further studies are warranted to evaluate protocols used, light sources, and incubation times, to determine how to make the therapy even more appealing to clinicians and patients alike.

References

[1] Jeffes EW, McCullough JL, Weinstein GD, et al. Photodynamic therapy of actinic keratoses with topical aminolevulinic acid hydrochloride and fluorescent blue light. J Am Acad Dermatol 2001;45:96–104.

[2] Stender IM. Treatment of human papilloma virus. In: Goldman MP, editor. Photodynamic therapy. Munich: Elsevier; 2005. p. 77–88.

[3] Bourke JF, Berth-Jones J, Hutchinson PE. Cryotherapy of common viral warts at intervals of 1, 2, and 3 weeks. Br J Dermatol 1995;132:433–6.

[4] Logan RA, Zachary CB. Outcome of carbondioxide laser therapy for persistent cutaneous viral warts. Br J Dermatol 1989;121:99.

[5] Tan OT, Hurwitz TM, Stafford TJ. Pulsed dye laser treatment of recalcitrant verrucae, a preliminary report. Lasers Surg Med 1993;13:127–37.

[6] Hirose R, Hori M, Shukuwa R, et al. Topical treatment of resistant warts with glutaraldehyde. J Dermatol 1994;21:248–53.

[7] Bunney MH, Nolan MW, Williams DA. An assessment of methods of treating viral warts by comparative treatment trials based on standard design. Br J Dermatol 1976;94:667–80.

[8] Halasz CL. Treatment of common warts using the infrared coagulator. J Dermatol Surg Oncol 1994;20:252–6.

[9] Brodell RT, Breadle DL. The treatment of palmar and plantar warts using natural alpha interferon and a needleless injector. Dermatol Surg 1995;21:213–8.

[10] James MP, Collier PM, Aherne W, et al. Histologic, pharmacologic and immunocytochemical effects of injection of bleomycin. J Am Acad Dermatol 1993;28:933–7.

[11] Shah KC, Patel RM, Umrigar DP. Dinitrochlorobenzene treatment of verrucae plana. J Dermatol 1991;18(11):639–42.

[12] Siegfried EC. Warts and molluscum contagiosum on children: an approach to therapy. Dermatol Ther 1997;2:51–67.

[13] Verbov J. How to manage warts. Arch Der Child 1999;80:97–9.

[14] Lewis EJ, Lam M, Crutchfield CE. An update on molluscum contagiosum. Cutis 1997;60:29–34.

[15] Husar K, Skerlev M. Molluscum contagiosum from infancy to maturity. Clin Dermatol 2002;20:170–2.

[16] Coldiron BM, Bergstresser PR. Prevalence and clinical spectrum of skin disease in patients infected with human immunodeficiency virus. Arch Dermatol 1989;125:357–61.

[17] Czelasta A, Yen-Moore A, Vander Straten M, et al. An overview of sexually transmitted diseases. Part III. Sexually transmitted diseases in HIV- infected patients. J Am Acad Dermatol 2000;43:409–32.

[18] Schwartz JJ, Myskowsk PL. Molluscum contagiosum in patients with human immunodeficiency virus infection: a review of twenty-seven patients. J Am Acad Dermatol 1992;27:583–8.

[19] Lowy DR. Molluscum contagiosum. In: Freedberg IM, Eisen AZ, Wolff K, et al, editors. Dermatology in general medicine. New York: The McGraw-Hill Companies; 1999. p. 2478–81.

[20] Matis WL, Triana A, Shapiro R, et al. Dermatologic findings associated with human immunodeficiency virus infection. J Am Acad Dermatol 1987;17 (5 Pt 1):746–51.

[21] Goodman DS, Teplitz ED, Wishner A, et al. Prevalence of cutaneous disease in patients with acquired immunodeficiency syndrome (AIDS) or AIDS-related complex. J Am Acad Dermatol 1987;17 (2 Pt 1):210–20.

[22] Epstein WL, et al. Viral antigens in human epidermal tumors: localization of an antigen to molluscum contagiosum. J Invest Dermatol 1963;40:51.

[23] Kwittken J. Molluscum contagiosum: some new histologic observations. Mt Sinai J Med 1980;47:583.

[24] Ammann R, Hunziker T, Braathen LR. Topical photodynamic therapy in verrucae. Dermatology 1995;191:346–7.

[25] Smetana Z, Malik Z, Orenstein A, et al. Treatment of viral infections with 5-aminolevulinic acid and light. Lasers Surg Med 1997;21:351–8.

[26] Stender IM, Na R, Fogh H, et al. Photodynamic therapy with 5-aminolevulinic acid or placebo for recalcitrant foot and hand warts: randomized double-blind trial. Clin Exp Dermatol 1999;24(3):154–9.

[27] Fabbrocini G, Costanzo M, Riccardo A, et al. Photodynamic therapy with topical 5-aminolevulinic acid for the treatment of plantar warts. J Photochem Photobiol B 2001;61:30–4.

[28] Stender IM, Lock-Andersen J, Wulf HC. Recalcitrant hand and foot warts successfully treated with photodynamic therapy with topical 5-aminolaevulinic acid: a pilot study. Clin Exp Dermatol 1999; 24:154–9.

[29] Mizuki D, Kaneko T, Hanada K. Successful treatment of topical photodynamic therapy using 5-aminolevulinic acid for plane warts. Br J Dermatol 2003; 149:1087–8.

[30] Smucler R, Jatsova E. Comparative study of aminolevulic acid photodynamic therapy plus pulsed dye laser versus pulsed dye laser alone in treatment of viral warts. Photomed Laser Surg 2005;23: 202–5.

[31] Gold MH. The use of ALA-PDT in the treatment of recalcitrant molluscum contagiosum in HIV/AIDS affected individuals. J Laser Surg Med 2003; 15:40.

ELSEVIER
SAUNDERS

DERMATOLOGIC
CLINICS

Dermatol Clin 25 (2007) 81–87

Methyl Aminolevulinate: Actinic Keratoses and Bowen's Disease

Colin A. Morton, MBChB, MD, FRCP

Forth Valley Dermatology Centre, Stirling Royal Infirmary, Stirling FK8 2AU, United Kingdom

Actinic keratoses (AK) and Bowen's disease can represent a management challenge for the dermatologist presented with a patient with multiple or large lesions, especially if arising in sites of high cosmetic importance. With both AK and Bowen's disease more prevalent in older age groups, and with a higher proportion of the population over 60 years of age, these epidermal dysplasias are set to become an ever more common reason for physician consultation. Increased numbers of long-term survivors from organ transplantation and prolonged immunosuppressant therapy also represent a patient group highly susceptible to nonmelanoma skin cancer. Patients in this group and those with more sensitive skin types and who have pursued extensive prolonged sunshine exposure can represent a particular management challenge with extensive areas of typically exposed skin demonstrating field cancerization and potential to develop a variety of nonmelanoma skin cancer. Topical PDT can be used to treat relatively large areas on a single visit, an advantage over standard focal therapies, such as cryotherapy or surgery. There is now the opportunity to treat subclinical lesions with the potential to slow and possibly prevent the development of new lesions. Reports of the efficacy of aminolevulinic acid (ALA) photodynamic

therapy (PDT) since 1990 indicate the potential of this therapy modality in the treatment of nonmelanoma skin cancer. The use of ALA-PDT has been reviewed elsewhere in this issue. This article evaluates the potential of topical methyl aminolevulinate (MAL) PDT for the treatment of AK and Bowen's disease.

Topical methyl aminolevulinate–photodynamic therapy for actinic keratoses and Bowen's disease: practical aspects

MAL, marketed as Metvix (Galderma, Paris, France and PhotoCure AS, Oslo, Norway) in Europe, Scandinavia, and Australia, is observed to have superior tissue selectivity and increased lipophilicity in comparison with nonesterified ALA. Topical MAL-PDT is approved but not yet marketed for AK in the United States, where it has Food and Drug Administration approval as Metvixia for nonhyperkeratotic AKs. On application MAL is converted by neoplastic tissue into photoactive porphyrins. Following illumination the photoactive porphyrins are converted to the higher energy triplet state, the energy being transferred then to oxygen molecules resulting in the formation of the cytotoxic free radicals and singlet oxygen critical to the PDT reaction.

To perform MAL-PDT it is advisable to prepare treatment sites by gentle removal of scale and overlying crust using either gauze soaked in saline with or without forceps, or a curette. It is important to note that such preparation is not intended to remove a significant amount of tissue as in typical curettage, and this preparation is done without any form of local anesthesia. MAL is applied for 3 hours (range 2.5–4 hours),

CAM has been an investigator for studies sponsored by Galderma, Paris, France and PhotoCure AS, Oslo, Norway, manufacturers of Metvix, methyl aminolevulinate, and received honoraria from participation in sponsored symposia. CAM has also received investigator support and honoraria from Schering AG, Berlin, Germany, and Phototherapeutics Ltd, Tamworth, UK.

E-mail address: colin.morton@fvah.scot.nhs.uk

preferably under occlusion, and treatment sites are then cleaned of excess cream before illumination with an appropriate light source. Although blue light can be used, most experience with MAL-PDT has been using red light to optimize tissue penetration. It is unclear the importance of this when treating AKs but certainly one comparison study of red and green light in Bowen's disease treated by ALA-PDT showed significant superiority of red over green [1] and it is presumed that a similar observation would have been noted had the comparison been with red and shorter wavelength blue light. It is common now to use an intense LED light source (634 ± 3 nm), such as the Aktilite (Galderma, Paris, France). Lesions are illuminated at an intensity of approximately 50 mW/cm^2 with a total dose of 37 J/cm^2 with the lamp positioned 50 to 80 mm from the skin. As a consequence of increased research experience, the protocol for treating AK in Europe now states that a single treatment is undertaken with assessment after 3 months for decision as to whether a repeat treatment is required. For Bowen's disease the license for MAL-PDT states that two treatments are undertaken 7 days apart with assessment for the need of further treatment made after 3 months. Following treatment patients can expect initial erythema and swelling of treated sites, which rapidly settles to be replaced by crusting, with resolution of these features after 4 to 6 weeks. Faint erythema may remain at treatment sites for a few months but high-quality cosmetic outcome is expected following topical MAL-PDT.

Topical methyl aminolevulinate–photodynamic therapy for actinic keratoses

Guidelines on the use of topical PDT published in 2002 supported the use of PDT for the treatment of nonhyperkeratotic AK on the face and scalp. Much of the evidence for this recommendation was on the basis of ALA-PDT studies [2]. The evidence to support the use of MAL-PDT for AK is reviewed next and summarized in Table 1.

There have been five major studies of the efficacy of MAL-PDT in the treatment of AKs. In the first multicenter study performed in Europe [3], 699 AKs in 193 patients received treatment (92% on face and scalp; 93% of lesions were thin or moderately thick). There was similar efficacy between a single treatment with MAL-PDT in comparison with two freeze-thaw cycles of cryotherapy. Three months after last treatment

75% of thin (slightly palpable AKs) and 66% of moderate thickness AKs had cleared with PDT compared with 80% and 71%, respectively, in the cryotherapy group. Excellent or good cosmetic outcome was reported in 96% of patients treated with MAL-PDT compared with 80% of those receiving cryotherapy, a significant difference in favor of PDT.

In a second multicenter study performed in Australia [4], MAL-PDT was repeated after 7 days and this double treatment was compared with a single treatment with cryotherapy as typically performed by the dermatologists involved in the study. Three months following last treatment of the 855 lesions studied, 91% of those lesions treated with MAL-PDT had cleared, significantly superior to the 68% of AK treated with cryotherapy and the 30% placebo response. Excellent cosmetic outcome was reported in 84% of patients treated with MAL-PDT (excellent or good in 98%) in comparison with 51% for cryotherapy.

In a third multicenter randomized double-blind study performed in the United States, 80 patients with 502 AK were studied [5]. PDT was undertaken with a repeat at 1 week, with lesion clearance after PDT of 89% in comparison with 38% placebo response. Excellent or good cosmesis was noted in 97% of patients treated with MAL-PDT. The placebo response has interested some observers but it should be recalled that a number of lesions studied are very subtle, where lesion preparation may have been sufficient to achieve apparent clearing of lesions 3 month out. It is also recognized that up to 25% of AK may undergo spontaneous regression.

A recent comparison of two treatment regimes with MAL-PDT has revolutionized the way that topical MAL-PDT is delivered in Europe and confirmed the efficacy of the red LED light sources now in routine use [6]. In a study of 211 patients with 413 thin or moderate AK on the face and scalp, patients were randomized to receive either a single treatment with MAL-PDT repeated at 3 months only if partial clinical response was observed, compared with the standard protocol of two treatments with MAL-PDT 7 days apart with assessment of efficacy at 3 months. An initial MAL-PDT treatment for these thin and moderate AK led to a clearance of 81% of lesions (93% of thin lesions). A second treatment in only those lesions requiring it brought the clearance rate to 92%, whereas the double treatment with MAL-PDT 7 days apart cleared 87% of lesions. On the

Table 1
Main clinical trials of methyl aminolevulinate—photodynamic therapy in actinic keratoses

Study design	Design	Study size	Follow-up	Overall clearance	Cosmesis
MAL-PDT (×1) vs cryotherapy (2 freeze cycle) [3]	Randomized, multicentre	193 patients 699 AK (367 treated by MAL-PDT)	12 wk	MAL-PDT–69% Cryotherapy–75%	MAL-PDT significantly superior to cryotherapy (good or excellent in 96% for PDT and 81% for cryotherapy)
MAL-PDT (×2ª) vs placebo-PDT (×2ª) vs cryotherapy (1 freeze cycle) [4]	Randomized, placebo-controlled, multicentre	200 patients 763 AK (295 treated by MAL-PDT)	12 wk	MAL-PDT–91% Placebo-PDT–30% Cryotherapy–68%	MAL-PDT significantly superior to cryotherapy (excellent in 81% for PDT, 98% combined score for good and excellent, and 51% for cryotherapy)
MAL-PDT (×2ª) vs placebo PDT(×2ª) [5]	Randomized, placebo-controlled, multicentre	80 patients 502 lesions (260 treated by MAL-PDT)	12 wk	MAL-PDT–89% Placebo-PDT–38%	Excellent or good cosmetic outcome reported in 97% of patients treated with MAL-PDT
Comparison: MAL-PDT ×1 repeated if necessary at 3 mo vs MAL-PDT (×2ª) [6]	Randomized, multicentre	211 patients 400 AK	12 wk after last treatment	MAL-PDT ×1, repeated if necessary–92% (81% after first treatment) MAL-PDT (×2ª) –87%	Excellent cosmetic outcome reported in >75% of treatment sites in each group
MAL-PDT (×1) vs cryotherapy (2 freeze cycle), repeat at 12 wk, if required	Randomized, intra-individual, multicentre	119 patients 1505 AK	12 wk after last treatment	MAL-PDT–89% (84% after one treatment) Cryotherapy–86% (75% after one treatment)	MAL-PDT significantly superior to cryotherapy (excellent in 71% for PDT and 57% for cryotherapy)
MAL-PDT (×2ª) vs 2 × placebo PDT (×2ª) [8]	Randomized, placebo controlled, intra-individual	17 patients	16 wk	MAL-PDT treated AK clear in 13/17 patients. partial response in 3 patients Placebo PDT no sites cleared	MAL-PDT cosmetic outcome rated uniformly as excellent

ª Two treatments 7 days apart.

basis of this study the protocol for MAL-PDT in Europe has now changed, saving unnecessary treatment and expense.

In a recently completed 24-week, multicenter, randomized, intraindividual (right-left) study [7], 119 recruited subjects with 1505 AK received both one treatment session of MAL-PDT, again with the LED light sources, and a double freeze-thaw cryotherapy, repeated after 3 months if incomplete response; the treatments were randomly allocated to either side of the face or scalp. At week 12, treatment with MAL-PDT resulted in significantly larger rate of cured lesions relative to cryotherapy (84.4% versus 74.5%), with a similar cure rate at week 24 (89.1% for MAL-PDT versus 86.1% for cryotherapy). Results for subject and investigator preferences and cosmetic outcome favored MAL-PDT.

A further randomized, placebo-controlled, double-blind study of the use of MAL-PDT in organ transplant recipients assessed the response of AK in 17 patients each with two suitable sites identified, with a follow-up at 4 months [8]. Two MAL-PDT treatments 7 days apart were compared with placebo PDT. There was lesion clearing in 13 of the 17 sites with a partial response in a further three and no change in the remaining one patient. There was no reduction in size or number of lesions in the sites treated by placebo PDT. This study has suggested the potential of MAL-PDT in a group of patients particularly prone to actinic damage and to the hazards of field cancerization.

An open intrapatient randomized trial has also explored the potential of MAL-PDT to prevent new lesions from forming [9]. The study, of 27 renal transplant recipients with AKs and other skin lesions in two contralateral sites, received PDT only to one area. The mean time to the occurrence of a new lesion was significantly longer (9.6 months) compared with the control sites (6.8 months). After 12 months, 62% of treated sites were free from new lesions compared with only 35% of control sites.

The place of methyl aminolevulinate–photodynamic therapy for the treatment of actinic keratoses

The reviewed studies confirm high efficacy for the use of MAL-PDT for thin and moderate-thickness AK. The superior cosmetic outcome is of particular importance as a therapy for AK, in view of their development typically on visible cosmetically sensitive body sites. Although erythema and swelling occur following PDT, the profile of response of a short-term intense reaction settling to low-grade erythema with or without crusting seems more acceptable than alternative current therapies.

It should be noted that in those studies that have looked at the treatment of thicker lesions (eg, the European multicenter study [3]), a single treatment with MAL-PDT still achieved clearance of 52% of lesions. Most studies have focused on the use of MAL-PDT for treatment of lesions only on the face and scalp. There is no reason to expect that response rates with MAL-PDT for acral lesions is inferior to the observed experience with ALA-PDT where, although response rates are typically lower, a beneficial clinical response can be achieved with the potential added benefit of treating sites of field cancerization.

The potential for MAL-PDT in immunosuppressed patients including organ transplant recipients is also encouraging, although further studies are required. If the observation that MAL-PDT can delay the development of new AK and other nonmelanoma skin cancer is confirmed with larger studies, the potential to reduce, in particular, the number of squamous cell carcinomas could justify preventative routine PDT in susceptible individuals.

Methyl aminolevulinate–photodynamic therapy in Bowen's disease

Bowen's disease has been widely proposed as an indication for topical PDT with several studies confirming the efficacy of ALA-PDT including randomized comparison studies demonstrating the superiority of PDT to topical 5-fluorouracil in a two center study and the equivalence of topical PDT to cryotherapy in a noninferiority study also undertaken in the same center [10,11].

Recently, a large multicenter study has been completed comparing MAL-PDT with clinician's choice of either cryotherapy or topical 5-fluorouracil. A total of 225 patients with 275 lesions were entered into the study with 111 lesions treated with MAL-PDT. MAL-PDT was delivered as two treatments performed 7 days apart with a repeat cycle of treatment after 3 months if necessary [12]. Cryotherapy was performed as a single freeze-thaw cycle to achieve an ice field that persisted for a minimum of 20 seconds and topical 5-fluorouracil was applied once daily for 1 week and then twice daily for 3 weeks.

Cryotherapy and topical 5-fluorouracil were also repeated after 3 months if required. Three months after the last treatment, MAL-PDT achieved clearance of 93% of lesions in comparison with 86% and 83% for cryotherapy and topical 5-fluorouracil, respectively. Cosmetic outcome at 3 months was reported as good or excellent for 94% of patients receiving PDT in comparison with 66% for cryotherapy and 76% for 5-fluorouracil. After 12 months of follow-up, the estimated sustained lesion complete response rate with MAL-PDT was superior to cryotherapy (80% versus 67%, $P = .047$), and better than with 5-fluorouracil (80% versus 69%, $P = .19$). Recurrence rates for 24 months have recently been presented with an 18% rate comparable with 23% for cryotherapy and 21% for 5-fluorouracil [13]. As a consequence of these results topical MAL-PDT has recently been approved in most European countries for the treatment of Bowen's disease, using a protocol with dosimetry as with MAL-PDT for AK, but with two treatments 7 days apart, repeated at 3 months, if required.

Data concerning longer-term clearance rates following standard treatments for Bowen's disease are limited, but in one retrospective study of 617 patients with Bowen's disease [14] relapse rates (>5 years) of 34% for cryotherapy, 19% for curettage, 14% for 5-fluorouracil, 6% for radiotherapy, and 5% for surgery were observed. With a 64-month recurrence rate of 17% noted in our long-term follow-up of ALA-PDT, it would be surprising if the recurrence rate profile was not similar with MAL-PDT [15]. For Bowen's disease, topical PDT can be viewed as having an acceptable long-term efficacy, comparable with more established therapies.

The potential of photodynamic therapy in Bowen's disease

MAL-PDT is confirmed as an effective therapy in Bowen's disease. Although no direct comparison with ALA formulations has been undertaken, MAL-PDT seems to achieve clearance rates similar to ALA-PDT. It is reasonable to assume that the top evidence ratings awarded in clinical guidelines also apply to MAL-PDT [2]. Topical PDT for Bowen's disease as a tissue-sparing, non-invasive therapy with high efficacy and good tolerability is well suited for treatment of Bowen's disease, which often appears in slow-healing sites.

Topical PDT seems to be a particular option for the treatment of large and multiple patches of Bowen's disease [16]. An initial clearance rate following ALA-PDT for 40 large, 20- to 55-mm diameter lesions achieved clearance after one to three treatments of 88% falling to 78% by 12 months. In the same study, 10 patients with 45 patches of Bowen's disease saw an overall clearance rate with PDT of 89% after 12 months.

Case reports and series attest to the beneficial use of topical PDT in rarer, but therapeutically challenging presentations of Bowen's disease. A patient with Bowen's disease of the nail bed was successfully treated, following a partial nail evulsion, by four cycles of PDT, initially with ALA-PDT, then MAL-PDT [17].

Perianal squamous cell carcinoma in situ has been successfully treated in three cases reported using systemic photosensitizer, porfimer sodium [18], but no publications of the use of topically applied agents have been identified. In my experience with two patients, partial (50%–80%) clearing perianally was achieved, but treatment at the anal margin proved unsuccessful.

In view of the predilection for Bowen's disease to develop on the lower leg, especially in women, topical PDT is proposed as a good treatment option for this site, where tissue preservation, rapid healing, and good cosmesis are achievable [19].

Organ transplant recipients with confirmed AK or Bowen's disease received ALA-PDT and demonstrated initial clinical response at a level to match the response of immunocompetent controls with the same diagnoses. An initial cure rate at 4 weeks of 86% reduced to 68% after 12 weeks, then 48% by 12 weeks. Because host immune responses contribute to the clearance of tumors, including clearance of residual tumor cells, reduced response of immunocompromised patients to such therapies as PDT is not surprising, but a clinically significant contribution to the management of this patient group is encouraging and further studies with MAL-PDT, beyond AK [8], are awaited [20].

Erythroplasia of Queyrat can respond to topical PDT, but the case reports of the use of ALA-PDT urge caution regarding ensuring sustained response by careful follow-up [21,22]. Bowenoid papulosis, the rare condition characterized by single or multiple red-brown warty papules in the anogenital area and with histology similar to Bowen's disease, has also been reported to respond to ALA-PDT [23].

Can topical PDT using MAL be effective for invasive squamous cell carcinoma? Studies using

MAL are awaited, but three open-label studies have described the use of ALA-PDT in squamous cell carcinoma, with initial complete response rates of 54% to 100% for superficial lesions, but with recurrence rates of up to 69% (mean 24%, 12 of 49, after 3–47 months). Only 40% (4 of 10) of nodular squamous cell carcinomas remained clear after 12 to 36 months [24–26]. Although ALA-PDT has shown efficacy, the relatively high recurrence rates for a potentially metastatic lesion restricts its use and this is not a licensed indication for topical PDT.

Methyl aminolevulinate–photodynamic therapy for actinic keratoses and Bowen's disease: adverse events

No particular adverse events particular to AK and Bowen's disease have been observed but the use of MAL-PDT does seem less painful than ALA, at least in a normal skin model [27]. It is common for patients to experience some pain or discomfort, typically described as a burning or prickling sensation, but no local anesthesia was necessary in the MAL-PDT studies reviewed previously. Experience from a busy PDT clinic suggests that multiple face and scalp AK can be expected to be more uncomfortable to treat than, for example, a patch of Bowen's disease on the shin. It is important, however, always to consider the risk-benefit profile for any treatment and that whereas the risk of discomfort is greater for treating large areas of actinic damage on the face, the expected benefit to the patient is greater, where one can anticipate more rapid healing and superior cosmetic outcome to standard therapy. Moreover, as a physician-controlled therapy, it is feasible in patients where particular discomfort might be anticipated to provide local anesthesia or analgesia. In my clinical practice, I routinely use a cool air device that, if preferred, the patient can hold and direct the cool air to the site of particular discomfort. Others use simple sprayed cold water to provide relief or ordinary cool air fans. The use of topical anesthesia has been disappointing when studied, although is seems to offer beneficial relief to certain patients. The observation of hyperpigmentation and hypopigmentation following topical MAL-PDT is uncommon.

Summary

The studies reviewed demonstrate a confirmed high efficacy with good cosmetic outcome associated with the use of topical MAL-PDT for the treatment of nonhyperkeratotic AK and Bowen's disease. The option of an area-wide therapy for AK, which may help reduce and even prevent a proportion of new lesions, is encouraging, with the added advantage of the high-quality cosmetic outcome to be expected when treating sites that are usually on exposed areas. Prolonged follow-up is typically lacking for treatments of AK, because it is difficult to monitor individuals with the added need to accommodate for new lesion development and spontaneous clearance of others during follow-up. High efficacy of MAL-PDT in Bowen's disease has now been confirmed and prolonged follow-up out to 24 months is reassuring, with relapse rates slightly lower (although not statistically) than cryotherapy and topical 5-fluorouracil.

There is now good evidence to suggest that MAL-PDT be considered a first-line option in the treatment of AK and Bowen's disease, especially if multiple, large, or in cosmetically sensitive sites. This physician-controlled treatment can be delivered within a half-day visit to a clinic, and it is convenient to patients especially considering the typically older age group of individual who develop extensive AK and Bowen's disease. The high standard of cosmetic outcome following PDT has been an added bonus of this therapy with evidence of photorejuvenation following PDT suggesting that yet further benefits from MAL-PDT might be achievable, although publication of specific studies of photorejuvenation with MAL-PDT are awaited.

References

[1] Morton CA, Whitehurst C, Moore JV, et al. Comparison of red and green light in the treatment of Bowen's disease by photodynamic therapy. Br J Dermatol 2000;143:767–72.

[2] Morton CA, Brown SB, Collins C, et al. Guidelines for topical photodynamic therapy: report of a workshop of the British Photodermatology Group. Br J Dermatol 2002;146:552–67.

[3] Szeimies RM, Karrer S, Radakovic-Fijan S, et al. Photodynamic therapy using topical methyl 5-aminolevulinate compared with cryotherapy for actinic keratosis: a prospective, randomized study. J Am Acad Dermatol 2002;47:258–62.

[4] Freeman M, Vinciullo C, Francis D, et al. A comparison of photodynamic therapy using topical methyl aminolevulinate (Metvix) with single cycle cryotherapy in patients with actinic keratosis: a prospective, randomized study. J Dermatol Treat 2003; 14:99–106.

[5] Pariser DM, Lowe NJ, Stewart DM, et al. Yamauchi PS. Photodynamic therapy with topical methyl aminolevulinate for actinic keratosis: results of a prospective randomised multicenter trial. J Am Acad Dermatol 2003;48:227–32.

[6] Tarstedt M, Rosdahl I, Berne B, et al. A randomized multicenter study to compare two treatment regimens of topical methyl aminolevulinate (Metvix)-PDT in actinic keratosis of the face and scalp. Acta Derm Venereol 2005;85:1–5.

[7] Morton CA, Campbell S, Gupta G, et al. Intra-individual, right-left comparison of topical methyl aminolevulinate photodynamic therapy (MAL-PDT) and cryotherapy in subjects with actinic keratoses: a multicentre, randomized controlled study. Br J Dermatol 2006;155:1029–36.

[8] Dragieva G, Prinz BM, Hafner J, et al. A randomized controlled clinical trial of topical photodynamic therapy with methyl aminolaevulinate in the treatment of actinic keratoses in transplant recipients. Br J Dermatol 2004;151:196–200.

[9] Wulf HC, Pavel S, Stender I, et al. Topical photodynamic therapy for prevention of new skin lesions in renal transplant recipients. Acta Derm Venereol 2006;86:25–8.

[10] Salim A, Leman JA, McColl JH, et al. Randomized comparison of photodynamic therapy with topical 5-fluorouracil in Bowen's disease. Br J Dermatol 2003;148:539–43.

[11] Morton CA, Whitehurst C, Moseley H, et al. Comparison of photodynamic therapy with cryotherapy in the treatment of Bowen's disease. Br J Dermatol 1996;135:766–71.

[12] Morton C, Horn M, Leman J, et al. Comparison of topical methyl aminolevulinate photodynamic therapy with cryotherapy of fluorouracil for treatment of squamous cell carcinoma in-situ. Arch Dermatol 2006;142:729–35.

[13] Morton C, Horn M, Leman J, et al. A 24-month update of a placebo controlled European study comparing MAL-PDT with cryotherapy and 5-fluorouracil in patients with Bowen's Disease. J Eur Acad Dermatol Venereol 2005;19(Suppl 2): 237–1.

[14] Thestrup-Pedersen K, Ravnborg L, Reymann F, et al. A description of the disease in 617 patients. Acta Derm Venereol 1988;68:236–9.

[15] Leman JA, Mackie RM, Morton CA. Recurrence rates following aminolaevulinic acid- photodynamic therapy for intra-epidermal squamous cell carcinoma compare favourably with outcome following conventional modalities. Br J Dermatol 2002; 147(Suppl 62):35.

[16] Morton CA, Whitehurst C, McColl JH, et al. Photodynamic therapy for large or multiple patches of Bowen's disease and basal cell carcinoma. Arch Dermatol 2001;137:319–24.

[17] Tan B, Sinclair R, Foley P. Photodynamic therapy for subungual Bowen's disease. Australas J Dermatol 2004;45:172–4.

[18] Petrelli NJ, Cebollero JA, Rodriguez-Bigas M, et al. Photodynamic therapy in the management of neoplasms of the perianal skin. Arch Surg 1992;127: 1436–8.

[19] Ball SB, Dawber RPR. Treatment of cutaneous Bowen's disease with particular emphasis on the problem of lower leg lesions. Australas J Dermatol 1998;39:63–70.

[20] Dragieva G, Hafner J, Dummer R, et al. Topical photodynamic therapy in the treatment of actinic keratoses and Bowens disease in transplant recipients. Transplantation 2004;77:115–21.

[21] Stables GI, Stringer MR, Robinson DJ, et al. Erythroplasia of Queyrat treated by topical aminolaevulinic acid photodynamic therapy. Br J Dermatol 1999;140:514–7.

[22] Varma S, Holt PJA, Anstey AV. Erythroplasia of Queyrat treated by topical aminolaevulinic acid photodynamic therapy: a cautionary tale. Br J Dermatol 2000;142:825–6.

[23] Yang CH, Lee JC, Chen CH, et al. Photodynamic therapy for bowenoid papulosis using a novel incoherent light-emitting diode device. Br J Dermatol 2003;149:1297–8.

[24] Fink-Puches R, Soyer HP, Hofer A, et al. Long-term follow-up and histological changes of superficial nonmelanoma skin cancers treated with topical delta-aminolevulinic acid photodynamic therapy. Arch Dermatol 1998;134:821–6.

[25] Calzavara-Pinton PG. Repetitive photodynamic therapy with topical delta-aminolaevulinic acid as an appropriate approach to the routine treatment of superficial non-melanoma skin tumours. J Photochem Photobiol B 1995;29:53–7.

[26] Fritsch C, Goerz G, Ruzicka T. Photodynamic therapy in dermatology. Arch Dermatol 1998;134: 207–14.

[27] Wiegell SR, Stender IM, Na R, et al. Pain associated with photodynamic therapy using 5-aminolevulinic acid or 5-aminolevulinic acid methylester on tape-stripped normal skin. Arch Dermatol 2003;139:1173–7.

ELSEVIER
SAUNDERS

Dermatol Clin 25 (2007) 89–94

DERMATOLOGIC
CLINICS

Methyl Aminolevulinate-photodynamic Therapy for Basal Cell Carcinoma

Rolf-Markus Szeimies, MD, PhD

Department of Dermatology, Regensburg University Hospital, Franz-Josef-Strauss-Allee 11,
D-93053 Regensburg, Germany

Basal cell carcinomas (BCCs) are the commonest malignant tumors of the skin, arising from the basal cells of the epidermis. They are mainly located in sun-exposed areas like the face, the neck region, upper extremities, and the trunk and then rarely metastasize. Treatment of BCCs should be chosen according to clinical type, tumor size, and location. Because of the limited penetration of red light into tissue, tumor thickness is a determinant response parameter of BCCs to photodynamic therapy (PDT) with methyl aminolevulinate (MAL) (Metvix, Galderma, Paris, France) in combination with red light (Aktilite, Galderma), and should not exceed 2 to 3 mm to achieve complete destruction [1]. Nodular BCCs with vertical growth and greater thickness should be preferentially treated by surgery because treatment of nodular BCCs by single aminolevulinate acid (ALA) PDT has resulted in low average cure rates. Better results by far are achieved using MAL-PDT (possibly because of higher lipophilicity, more rapid skin penetration, and higher selectivity [2]) but also because of regular lesion preparation (debulking) before PDT.

In addition, pigmented BCCs do not allow an optimal penetration of the light and should not be treated with PDT. This restriction is also suggested for sclerosing BCCs with diffuse infiltrating and unpredictable borders. Superficial BCCs usually occur on the trunk and are often multiple. A large number of treatment modalities exist, especially for single superficial BCCs (eg, excisional surgery, curettage and electrocautery, cryotherapy, immune response modifiers, cytotoxic agents, or radiotherapy). In the treatment of multiple lesions (eg, in the case of basal cell nevus syndrome or in immunosuppressed patients after organ transplantation), however, PDT has the potential of becoming a first-line therapy with an excellent cosmesis but without complications like scar formation, requirement for grafts, need of multiple treatments, or pigmentary changes [2].

These conclusions are drawn from extensive studies in past years using MAL-PDT for both nodular and superficial BCCs (Tables 1 and 2).

Nodular basal cell carcinoma

Intravenously applied photosensitizers like sodium porfimer [3], verteporfin [4], and mTHPC [5] have demonstrated response rates of between 78% and 92% for nodular BCC. Phototoxicity and lack of lesion selectivity, however, has limited their development. With topical PDT for nodular BCC, delivery of sufficient amounts of photosensitizer and light to the full depth of the lesion is critical. Topical MAL has been shown effectively to penetrate into thick nodular BCC lesions [6]. MAL has superior tissue penetration over ALA because of its decreased charge and increased lipophilicity [6], although there is so far no direct comparison between both drugs in clinical studies of nodular BCC. In PDT for nodular BCC greater than 2 mm in thickness, response may be enhanced by debulking the tumor before treatment, with the retreatment of lesions also possible if necessary (normally repetition of treatment is recommended within 7–10 days). Table 1 shows the main clinical trials of topical MAL-PDT in nodular BCC.

E-mail address: rolf-markus.szeimies@klinik.
uni-regensburg.de

Table 1
Main clinical trials of topical methyl aminolevulinate-photodynamic therapy in nodular basal cell carcinoma

Study	Design	Study size	Dosage regimen	Results (PP population)
MAL-PDT [17]	Retrospective study	189 nBCC lesions Follow up: 24–48 mo	1 × MAL-PDT (lesion preparation[a])	3-mo lesion CR: 89% 35-mo recurrence rates were 7% thin nBCC and 14% thick nBCC
MAL-PDT difficult-to-treat BCC (European trial) [7]	Open-label study	40 nBCC lesions (38 sBCC lesions) Follow-up: 60 mo	2 × MAL-PDT, retreated after 3 mo where necessary (lesion preparation)	3-mo lesion CR: 87% 60-mo recurrence rate 18%
MAL-PDT vs surgery [9]	Multicenter, randomized, open-label study	101 patients 110 lesions (56 treated with MAL-PDT) Follow-up: 60 mo	2 × MAL-PDT (7 d apart) vs surgical excision (lesion preparation)	3-mo lesion CR: MAL-PDT (91%) similar to surgery (98%) 60-mo recurrence rates: MAL-PDT 14% vs surgery 4%. Recurrence rates for MAL-PDT at 60 mo the same as at 36 mo Excellent or good cosmetic outcome reported in 82% of patients treated with MAL-PDT vs 33% for surgery after 3 mo
MAL-PDT vs placebo PDT (US trial) [10]	Randomized, placebo-controlled double-blind study	65 patients 80 lesions (41 treated with MAL-PDT) Follow-up: 3 mo	2 × MAL-PDT (7 d apart) retreated after 3 mo where necessary vs placebo PDT (lesion preparation)	6-mo lesion CR (clinical and histologic): MAL-PDT (82% and 79%, respectively) vs placebo (49 and 35%, respectively) Excellent or good cosmetic outcome reported in 92% of patients treated with MAL-PDT 75% of patients found MAL-PDT better than (60%) or equal to (15%) previous therapy
MAL-PDT vs placebo PDT (Australian trial) [11]	Randomized, placebo-controlled double-blind study	66 patients 70 lesions (34 treated with MAL-PDT) Follow-up: 6 mo	2 × MAL-PDT (7 d apart) retreated after 3 mo where necessary vs placebo PDT (lesion preparation)	6-mo lesion CR (histologically controlled): MAL-PDT (73%) >placebo PDT (21%) Excellent or good cosmetic outcome reported in 95% of patients treated with MAL-PDT

(continued on next page)

Table 1 (*continued*)

Study	Design	Study size	Dosage regimen	Results (PP population)
MAL-PDT high-risk BCC (Australian trial) [8]	Open-label study	49 nBCC lesions (80 sBCC lesions) Follow-up: 48 mo	2 × MAL-PDT, retreated after 3 mo where necessary (lesion preparation)	3-mo lesion CR: 94% 48-mo recurrence rate 30%

Abbreviations: BCC, basal cell carcinoma; CR, complete remission; MAL, methyl aminolevulinate; nBCC, nodular basal cell carcinoma; PDT, photodynamic therapy; sBCC, superficial basal cell carcinoma.

[a] Lesion preparation, depending on the nature and thickness of the tumor, can be gentle removal of surface to debulking the center of the tumor within the margins.

Modified from Braathen LR, Szeimies RM, Basset-Seguin N, et al. Guidelines on the use of photodynamic therapy (PDT) for non-melanoma skin cancer—an international consensus. J Am Acad Dermatol, in press.

The strongest evidence for topical MAL-PDT in nodular BCC comes from five phase III studies in which a total of 220 nodular BCC lesions were treated [7–11]. A number of previous small open-label PDT studies revealed similar findings and support these data. Efficacy is constantly high, with 3-month complete response rates of 73% to 94% with MAL-PDT. Studies with histologic confirmation have set the reliability of efficacy data (73% and 79%) [10,11]. Horn and coworkers [7] and Vinciullo and coworkers [8] specifically studied the use of MAL-PDT in difficult-to-treat and high-risk cases and still found 3-month response rates of 87% and 94%, respectively. Former studies with ALA report variable efficacy (eg, 92% [12,13], 61% [14], and 64% [15]). Those lower rates may be caused by differences in lesion preparation and the use of nonstandardized light sources. In addition, the poorer penetration of ALA into nodular BCC may also contribute to lower efficacy compared with MAL [16].

A 5-year recurrence rate of 14% has been found in patients who participated in a phase III study of MAL-PDT for nodular BCC [9]. This rate is the same as at 36 months (ie, there were no further recurrences between 36 and 60 months after treatment), showing that MAL-PDT seems to remain effective in the longer term. For difficult-to-treat nodular BCC, recurrence rates at 48 to 60 months of follow-up vary from 18% to 30% [4,7,8,16]. In a retrospective study of patients receiving MAL-PDT for the treatment of nodular BCC, recurrence rates of 7% and 14% for thin and thick nodular BCC lesions were reported at a median 35-months follow-up [17]. This suggests that thin nodular BCC may be particularly responsive to MAL-PDT, although thickness of nodular BCC has not specifically been assessed in other trials. Thin nodular BCC are also likely to require less lesion preparation and may be best suited to treatment by topical PDT.

MAL-PDT has been compared with the gold standard approach of surgery for nodular BCC [9]. MAL-PDT provided a 3-month response rate noninferior to surgery (91% compared with 98% for surgery), and a 60-month recurrence rate of 14% compared with 4% for surgery [16].

MAL-PDT for nodular BCC is generally well tolerated, with predictable, transient, and manageable pain and erythema in most patients. Cosmetic outcomes with PDT in nodular BCC are generally very impressive, quoted as "excellent" or "good" in 82% to 95% of patients [7–11, 13,17,18]. Cosmetic outcome with PDT was found to be superior to cryotherapy [18] and surgery [9]. Cosmetic outcome with MAL-PDT was impressive even when the populations specifically included patients with lesions in cosmetically sensitive areas [7,8], with continued improvements seen in the long term. Nodular BCC lesions of less than 2 mm thick located outside the risk zone are considered low-risk tumors and their treatment should offer both optimal efficacy and cosmetic outcome [16].

Because MAL-PDT has been developed for nodular BCC using a standardized protocol, lesion preparation, light source, and dose, and because MAL offers superior penetration into the lesion, the evidence supports the use of MAL rather than ALA for PDT of nodular BCC. MAL-PDT is approved for the treatment of nodular BCC in the European Union, Australia, New Zealand, and Brazil [16].

MAL-PDT is an effective treatment for nodular BCC, when compared with surgery, but offering the advantage of superior cosmetic outcome.

Superficial basal cell carcinoma

Initial efficacy for MAL-PDT in superficial BCC is also consistently high. Three-month clearance rates with MAL-PDT range from 80% (in

Table 2
Main clinical trials of topical methyl aminolevulinate-photodynamic therapy in superficial basal cell carcinoma

Study	Design	Study size	Dosage regimen	Results (PP population)
MAL-PDT [17]	Retrospective study	147 sBCC lesions Follow up: 24–48 mo	1 × MAL-PDT (lesion preparation)	3-mo lesion CR: 91% 9% relapse at 35 mo Excellent cosmetic outcomes reported in 79% of patients
MAL-PDT difficult-to-treat BCC (European trial) [7]	Open-label multicenter study	38 sBCC lesions (40 nBCC lesions) Follow-up: 60-mo	2 × MAL-PDT, retreated after 3 mo where necessary (lesion preparation)	3 month lesion CR (with histological control): 80% 60-mo recurrence rate: 38% (52% very larges sBCC lesions) Excellent or good cosmetic outcome (total study population [n+sBCC]) reported in 94% of patients at 24 mo
MAL-PDT high-risk BCC (Australian trial) [8]	Open-label multicenter study	80 sBCC lesions (49 nBCC lesions) Follow-up: 48-mo	2 × MAL-PDT, retreated after 3 mo where necessary (lesion preparation)	3-mo lesion CR: 93% 48 month recurrence rate: 18% Excellent or good cosmetic outcome (total study population [n+sBCC]) reported in 86% of patients at 24 mo
MAL-PDT vs cryotherapy [19]	Randomized multicenter study	118 patients 219 lesions (102 treated with MAL-PDT) Follow-up: 60-mo	1 × MAL-PDT vs 2 × cryotherapy Patients retreated with 2 × MAL-PDT (7 d apart) or 2 × cryotherapy where necessary after 3 mo (lesion preparation)	3-mo lesion CR: MAL-PDT (97%) similar to cryotherapy (95%) 60-mo recurrence rates: MAL-PDT 22% similar to cryotherapy 20%. Recurrence rates for MAL-PDT at 60-mo the same as at 36-mo Excellent or good cosmetic outcomes reported in 89% of patients with MAL-PDT vs 50% for cryotherapy after 3-mo

Abbreviations: BCC, basal cell carcinoma; CR, complete remission; MAL, methyl aminolevulinate; nBCC, nodular basal cell carcinoma; PDT, photodynamic therapy; sBCC, superficial basal cell carcinoma.

Modified from Braathen LR, Szeimies RM, Basset-Seguin N, et al. Guidelines on the use of photodynamic therapy (PDT) for non-melanoma skin cancer—an international consensus. J Am Acad Dermatol, in press.

complex cases, with recurrent or large lesions, or H-zone lesions) [7,8] to 97% in primary superficial BCC. These included controlled studies of MAL-PDT with histologic confirmation [7,8]. Smaller open studies with ALA-PDT also support these data, with initial clearance rates of 90% to 100% in several primary superficial BCC studies [16].

New approaches for treatment of BCC are required not only to demonstrate high efficacy,

but also long-term responses that are at least equivalent to standard therapeutic procedures. Five-year follow-up of a phase III study [16,19] suggests that recurrence with MAL-PDT is comparable with cryotherapy (22% for MAL-PDT versus 20% for cryotherapy at 60 months). Recurrence rates are even lower for lesions ≤1 cm in diameter (with a 36-month recurrence rate of only 6% [16]). The recurrence rate at 60 months was the same as at 36 months following treatment with MAL-PDT [16,19] (ie, there were no additional recurrences after 36 months). In difficult-to-treat populations investigated by Horn and coworkers [7] and Vinciullo and coworkers [8], 36-month recurrence rates of 15% and 31% have been reported. Although recurrence in difficult-to-treat superficial BCC is higher than in primary superficial BCC, MAL-PDT does show good efficacy and is a viable alternative when surgery is inappropriate or the patient or physician wishes to maintain an optimal cosmetic result.

PDT was overall well tolerated in these patients, with some pain and erythema experienced by most patients. Wang and coworkers [18] found BCC patients experienced similar levels of pain with PDT and cryotherapy.

Surgery is still considered to be the gold standard treatment for BCC. Patients may not be appropriate for surgery, however, in certain situations (eg, large lesions, unsuitability for invasive therapy, poor ability for wound care, high risk of disfigurement, poor vasculature, concomitant use of anticoagulants, immunosuppression, diabetes, or inadequate prior response to standard therapies). Postsurgical scarring is often seen, with keloid or dystrophic scarring particularly problematic on the trunk, a common site for superficial BCC. Because of the relatively low-risk nature of superficial BCC, scarring problems should be taken into consideration when choosing a suitable therapy. Therefore, PDT may offer significant advantages over surgical or other destructive techniques. In a randomized comparator study of MAL-PDT, cosmetic outcome was superior to cryotherapy at 3 months (89% versus 50% of patients rated as having "good" or "excellent" cosmetic outcome [19]). Similar results were seen in the smaller randomized study by Wang and coworkers [18], who reported "excellent" or "good" cosmetic outcomes in 93% versus 54% for ALA-PDT and cryotherapy, although these figures include both superficial BCC and nodular BCC. High cure rates with superior cosmetic outcome makes PDT particularly well suited for the treatment of large, extensive, and multiple lesions. Interestingly, Horn and coworkers [7] and Vinciullo and coworkers [8] found that cosmetic outcome improved over time in difficult-to-treat populations (complex cases, with recurrent or large lesions, or H-zone lesions) who might be expected to have poor cosmetic outcomes. In difficult-to-treat patients with either nodular BCC or superficial BCC treated with MAL-PDT, 76%

of patients had excellent or good cosmetic outcomes, rising to 94% after 24 months [7].

PDT offers advantages over other therapies for superficial BCC, with high efficacy coupled with excellent cosmetic outcomes that are superior to cryotherapy [16].

Although MAL-PDT has proved its efficacy in long-term follow-up studies to be at least as efficient as standard alternative treatments to surgery, mandatory indications for surgical treatment are different histologic subtypes like pigmented or sclerosing BCCs or BCCs located in the area of the facial embryonic fusion clefts and all BCCs thicker than 3 mm if no debulking procedure is performed before PDT.

References

[1] Morton CA, Brown SB, Collins S, et al. Guidelines for topical photodynamic therapy: report of a workshop of the British Photodermatology Group. Br J Dermatol 2002;146:552–67.

[2] Szeimies RM, Morton CA, Sidoroff A, et al. Photodynamic therapy for non-melanoma skin cancer. Acta Derm Venereol 2005;85:483–90.

[3] Wilson BD, Mang TS, Stoll H, et al. Photodynamic therapy for the treatment of basal cell carcinoma. Arch Dermatol 1992;128:1597–601.

[4] Lui H, Hobbs L, Tope WD, et al. Photodynamic therapy of multiple nonmelanoma skin cancers with verteporfin and red light-emitting diodes: two-year results evaluating tumor response and cosmetic outcomes. Arch Dermatol 2004;140:26–32.

[5] Baas P, Saarnak AE, Oppelaar H, et al. Photodynamic therapy with meta-tetrahydroxyphenylchlorin for basal cell carcinoma: a phase I/II study. Br J Dermatol 2001;145:75–8.

[6] Peng Q, Soler AM, Warloe T, et al. Selective distribution of porphyrins in skin thick basal cell carcinoma after topical application of methyl 5-aminolevulinate. J Photochem Photobiol B 2001; 62:140–5.

[7] Horn M, Wolf P, Wulf HC, et al. Topical methyl aminolevulinate photodynamic therapy in patients with basal cell carcinoma prone to complications and poor cosmetic outcome with conventional therapy. Br J Dermatol 2003;149:1242–9.

[8] Vinciullo C, Elliott T, Francis D, et al. Photodynamic therapy with topical aminlaevulinate for 'difficult-to-treat' basal cell carcinoma. Br J Dermatol 2005;152:765–72.

[9] Rhodes LE, de Rie M, Enstrom Y, et al. Photodynamic therapy using topical methyl aminolevulinate vs surgery for nodular basal cell carcinoma: results of a multicenter randomized prospective trial. Arch Dermatol 2004;140:17–23.

[10] Tope WD, Menter A, El-Azhary RA, et al. Comparison of topical methyl aminolevulinate photodynamic therapy versus placebo photodynamic therapy in nodular BCC. J Eur Acad Dermatol Venereol 2004;18:413–4.

[11] Foley P, Freeman M, Siller G, et al. MAL-PDT or placebo cream in nodular basal cell carcinoma: results of an Australian double blind randomized multicentre study [poster]. Presented at the International Skin Cancer Conference, Zurich, July 22–24, 2004.

[12] Soler AM, Warloe T, Tausjo J, et al. Photodynamic therapy by topical aminolevulinic acid, dimethylsulphoxide and curettage in nodular basal cell carcinoma: a one-year follow-up study. Acta Derm Venereol 1999;79:204–6.

[13] Thissen MR, Schroeter CA, Neumann HA. Photodynamic therapy with delta-aminolaevulinic acid for nodular basal cell carcinomas using a prior debulking technique. Br J Dermatol 2000;142:338–9.

[14] Calzavara-Pinton PG. Repetitive photodynamic therapy with topical delta-aminolaevulinic acid as an appropriate approach to the routine treatment of superficial non-melanoma skin tumours. J Photochem Photobiol B 1995;29:53–7.

[15] Svanberg K, Andersson T, Killander D, et al. Photodynamic therapy of non-melanoma malignant tumours of the skin using topical delta-amino levulinic acid sensitization and laser irradiation. Br J Dermatol 1994;130:743–51.

[16] Braathen LR, Szeimies RM, Basset-Seguin N, et al. Guidelines on the use of photodynamic therapy (PDT) for non-melanoma skin cancer— an international consensus. J Am Acad Dermatol, in press.

[17] Soler AM, Warloe T, Berner A, et al. A follow-up study of recurrence and cosmesis in completely responding superficial and nodular basal cell carcinomas treated with methyl 5-aminolaevulinate-based photodynamic therapy alone and with prior curettage. Br J Dermatol 2001;145:467–71.

[18] Wang I, Bendsoe N, Klinteberg CA, et al. Photodynamic therapy vs. cryosurgery of basal cell carcinomas: results of a phase III clinical trial. Br J Dermatol 2001;144:832–40.

[19] Basset-Seguin N, Ibbotson S, Emtestam L, et al. Photodynamic therapy using Metvix is as efficacious as cryotherapy in BCC, with better cosmetic results. J Eur Acad Dermatol Venereol 2004;18:412.

DERMATOLOGIC
CLINICS

Dermatol Clin 25 (2007) 95–100

Chemopreventative Thoughts for Photodynamic Therapy

Robert Bissonnette, MD

Innovaderm Research, 1851 Sherbrooke Street East, Suite 502, Montreal, QC H2K 4L5, Canada

Photodynamic therapy (PDT) combines the administration of a photosensitizer to its subsequent activation by light of the appropriate waveband [1]. Aminolevulinic acid (ALA) and methyl aminolevulinate (MAL) are currently the only two PDT drugs approved by the Food and Drug Administration for use in dermatology. These drugs are photosensitizer precursors or prodrugs because they need to be converted into porphyrins by intracellular enzymes to make cells sensitive to the activating visible light [2].

Both ALA and MAL are approved for the treatment of actinic keratoses (AK), which are precursors of squamous cell carcinoma (SCC). The spot treatments of AKs by either ALA or MAL-PDT can be considered as a skin cancer prevention modality because AKs are premalignant. The concept of chemoprevention of skin cancer by PDT has been recently expanded following the publication of a number of preclinical and clinical studies with large surface ALA- and MAL-PDT. These studies suggest that large surface application of ALA or MAL followed by light exposure does not only treat visible AK but can prevent the appearance of new AKs and skin cancer. This article reviews the use of large surface PDT with ALA or MAL as a skin cancer prevention modality.

Animal studies on prevention of skin cancer by photodynamic therapy

Prevention of actinic keratoses and squamous cell carcinoma using the hairless mouse model

The hairless mouse is the most frequently used animal model to study the chemopreventive potential of PDT [3]. These immunocompetent mice have very sparse hair and do not have to be shaved before UV exposure. When irradiated daily with UV radiation these mice exhibit visible AK after a few months of exposure [4]. The time required for development of AK varies according to the spectral output of the UV source, the frequency of exposure, and the daily UV fluence used. In experiments designed to study the ability of PDT to delay skin cancer appearance, groups of hairless mice are usually exposed to UV radiation from artificial sources 5 or 7 days per week. PDT is performed weekly and mice are also examined weekly for the presence of tumors. Tumors are mapped and any tumor of at least 1 mm and present for at least 2 consecutive weeks is counted as a UV-induced tumor. Histologic studies have shown that small tumors (less than 4 mm) are AK, whereas larger tumors are invasive SCC [3]. UV irradiation does not generate melanoma or basal cell carcinoma (BCC) in this animal model. Tumor-free survival curves are generated for mice exposed only to UV radiation and mice exposed to UV and treated weekly with PDT. These curves are analyzed statistically using the log-rank test.

The first animal study suggesting that large surface ALA-PDT could prevent the appearance of skin cancer was published in 1997 by Stender and coworkers [5]. They exposed groups of mice

Dr. Bissonnette received research funding from DUSA Pharmaceuticals and Photocure ASA. He also served as a consultant for Photocure ASA.

E-mail address: rbissonnette@innovaderm.ca

daily to either UV radiation only or UV radiation with concomitant weekly ALA-PDT. They showed that weekly ALA-PDT could delay the appearance of AK in mice chronically exposed to UV radiation. They observed a higher mortality rate and higher number of mice withdrawn because of large tumors, however, in groups of mice treated with ALA-PDT. At about the same time our group initiated studies with systemic ALA in the same mouse model [6]. Groups of mice were exposed daily to UV radiation and injected weekly with ALA followed by white light exposure, whereas other groups of mice were only exposed to UV radiation. These studies showed that weekly systemic ALA-PDT could delay the appearance of AK and skin cancer. An increase in mortality or an increase in large tumors was not observed in mice treated with ALA-PDT. The UV radiation source and the visible light source used in our experiments with systemic ALA were different from the ones used by Stender and coworkers [5] with topical ALA.

Our group [7] subsequently repeated the systemic ALA experiments and topical ALA experiments using UV and visible light sources similar to Stender and coworkers [5]. These studies showed that weekly topical ALA-PDT could delay the appearance of AK and SCC without any increase in mortality or incidence of large tumors. We also performed studies with the hairless mouse model using parameters and conditions that were as close as possible to the clinical use of ALA-PDT in North America. These experiments were conducted with the commercially available ALA solution Levulan (DUSA Pharmaceuticals, Wilmington, Massachusetts) and the Blu-U as the activating light source. These experiments also included groups of mice that were exposed to UV before the beginning of the ALA-PDT sessions. In all other skin cancer prevention experiments using the hairless mouse model, large surface PDT was initiated at the same time as UV exposure. In clinical practice, however, physicians always advise patients with multiple AKs to avoid sun exposure. Patients who undergo large surface ALA-PDT already have had most of their UV exposure in the years preceding PDT. These studies confirmed that weekly large surface ALA-PDT performed with the commercially available ALA and blue light source can delay the appearance of AK and SCC. This delay was observed when UV exposure and PDT were started at the same time and when UV exposure was performed before the beginning of weekly ALA-PDT sessions.

In another series of experiments we used the hairless mouse model to study the safety of weekly ALA-PDT sessions without exposure to UV radiation [8]. Hairless mice are very sensitive to the development of skin cancer following UVB, PUVA, or chemical carcinogen exposure [9]. ALA was applied weekly on the back of mice followed by exposure to blue light for a total of 10 months. Mice were observed for an additional 2 months. In all these experiments AK and SCC were never observed despite weekly ALA-PDT for 10 months.

Similar skin cancer prevention experiments in hairless mice were also conducted with MAL [10,11]. Weekly MAL-PDT was able to delay the appearance of AK and SCC in hairless mice. In these experiments groups of mice received MAL-PDT on only half the back to explore if the mechanism of action was mostly a local or systemic phenomenon. Delay in skin cancer appearance was only noted for the half-back that received MAL and light and not the half-back that received vehicle and light.

Prevention of basal cell carcinoma using the PTCH mouse model

Mutations in the PTCH gene has been shown to be present in patients with Gorlin's syndrome [12]. This gene codes for a transmembrane protein, which binds to smoothened, another cell membrane protein. When this binding does not take place smoothened is activated, which triggers a series of events leading to transformation. Mutations in the PTCH gene can generate an altered PTCH protein with a decreased binding affinity to smoothened, which contributes to the development of BCC. PTCH mutations have been identified not only in patients with basal cell nevus syndrome (Gorlin's syndrome) but also in sporadic BCCs. We have used the transgenic PTCH mouse to study the ability of PDT to prevent the appearance of BCC [13]. This mouse model develops microscopic BCCs when chronically exposed to UV [14].

A group of PTCH +/− mice was exposed daily to UV radiation for a period of 20 weeks and treated weekly with large surface MAL-PDT, whereas another group was only exposed to UV. Euthanasia was performed 8 weeks later and more than 2000 sections were cut and analyzed blindly for the presence of BCC. A total of 19 BCCs were found in mice exposed chronically to UV and not treated with MAL-PDT, whereas no BCC was found in mice exposed to UV and treated with

MAL-PDT. In addition to BCCs, two visible SCCs were present in mice exposed to UV and not treated with MAL-PDT as compared with none in the MAL-PDT–treated group. This experiment suggests that multiple large surface PDT also has the ability to prevent BCC.

Clinical studies on prevention of skin cancer by photodynamic therapy

Prevention of actinic keratoses and squamous cell carcinoma

Wulf and coworkers [15] used MAL-PDT (one session) to treat 5 cm^2 skin areas in 27 immunosuppressed transplant patients. MAL was applied for 3 hours followed by illumination with 75 J/cm^2 of 570 to 670 red light. A control area of the same size was left untreated. New AK lesions were noted after a mean of 9.6 months in the areas treated with MAL-PDT, whereas it took a mean of 6.8 months for new AK lesions to appear in control areas. Twelve months after PDT 63% of the MAL-PDT–treated areas were devoid of new AK, whereas only 35% of the control areas were devoid of new AKs.

De Graaf and coworkers [16] treated 45 immunosuppressed transplant patients with PDT on the forearms. Forty patients were randomized to either one or two PDT treatments on one forearm, whereas the first five patients were initially treated in a nonrandomized pilot study. Patients had to have at least a 5-year history of immunosuppression following an organ transplant and at least 10 keratotic lesions on both forearms and hands to be eligible. The authors did not try to differentiate between seborrheic keratoses, warts, and AK and included all lesions as keratotic skin lesions. One forearm and hand was randomized to be treated with ALA-PDT, whereas the other served as control area and remained untreated. All patients received an ALA-PDT session at baseline and about half received a second treatment at 6 months. ALA was compounded at 20% in a cream base and applied under occlusion with Tegaderm for 4 hours. Patients were exposed to 5.5 to 6 J/cm^2 of 400- to 450-nm light from a Philips HPM-10 light source. Lesions were not pretreated before ALA application. Patents were followed every 3 months for 2 years. Any lesion suspicious of SCC was biopsied to obtain histologic confirmation. Only histologically confirmed SCC was included in the analysis. A total of 25 SCC were observed on hands and forearms during the 2-year follow-up period. Altogether 15 of these SCC developed on the PDT-treated arm, whereas 10 developed on the control arm. The control arm had less SCC than the treated arm in 20% of patients, whereas the PDT-treated arm had less SCC than the control arm in 17.5% of patients. In the remaining patients there was no difference between the PDT-treated and the control arm. The number of new SCC on the treated arm as compared with the control arm was not statistically different. The number of new keratotic lesions was also evaluated at each visit. There was no reduction in keratotic lesions after PDT. There was no statistically significant difference in the number of new keratotic lesions between the control arm and the ALA-PDT–treated arm in terms of keratotic skin lesions.

In contrast, Dragieva and coworkers [17] treated with ALA-PDT 21 transplant patients and 20 control immunocompetent patients with multiple AKs. An area of 3 × 4 cm on average was treated once or twice (1 day apart) and patients were followed for 1 year. A total of 40 lesion fields of an average of 3 × 4 cm containing AK and four lesion fields of 1.6 × 2 cm with Bowen's disease were treated once or twice (1 day apart) and patients were followed for 1 year. A total of 32 lesional areas with AK and four areas with Bowen's disease in immunocompetent patients were also treated in the same manner. ALA at 20% in an oil in water emulsion was applied on the area to be treated and 5 mm of adjacent skin with occlusion. Five hours later the area was exposed to 75 J/cm^2 of red light from a Waldmann 1200 PDT illuminator. The overall complete response rates were 86%, 68%, and 48% at 4, 12, and 84 weeks, respectively. The cure rates were comparable for immunocompetent and immunosuppressed patients at week 4 but were lower in immunosuppressed patients at week 12 and 84. This study suggests that there might be differences between transplant patients with multiple AKs and immunocompetent patients with multiple AKs.

As opposed to Dragieva and coworkers [17] who showed an 86% complete response in AKs at 3 months, de Graaf and coworkers [16] showed no improvement in the number of keratotic lesions at 3 months after PDT. A number of factors may explain the difference in outcome between these two studies. In the de Graaf study [16] curettage was not performed before ALA application and half of the patients received only one ALA-PDT session. In addition, blue light was used instead of red light. In the de Graaf study only patients with a 5-year history of organ transplant with a history of previous skin cancer or at least 10 keratotic lesions were eligible and patients were treated only twice with ALA-PDT. It is possible ALA-PDT is more effective in preventing AK and SCC when the intervention is started at an earlier stage. In our hairless mouse experiments the delay in skin cancer appearance observed when ALA-PDT was started 8 weeks after the beginning of UV exposure was not as important as when ALA-PDT was started at the same time as UV-exposure. In a transplant patient population one or two ALA-PDT sessions might not be sufficient [18]. It is also well known that the response to ALA-PDT of AK located on the upper limbs is not as good as lesions located on the face, presumably because of decreased penetration through more hyperkeratotic lesions. In the de Graaf study [16] no lesion preparation was performed. Many physicians perform a mild curettage of hyperkeratotic AKs before application of ALA or MAL to enhance penetration and PDT response.

A multicenter, randomized study in transplant recipients is currently underway to assess the efficacy of multiple large surface MAL-PDT to prevent nonmelanoma skin cancer and AK [19]. A total of 81 patients with a minimum of two AK and a maximum of 10 skin lesions (AK, BCC, SCC in situ, or warts) in two symmetrical contralateral areas of the face, scalp extremities, neck, or trunk have been included in this study. One of these areas was treated with MAL-PDT at baseline, 3 months, 9 months, and 15 months, whereas lesions in the contralateral area were treated with standard therapy (mainly cryotherapy). PDT with 37 J/cm^2 of red light was performed 3 hours after MAL application. Lesions were prepared using a curette before MAL application. Efficacy assessment included the number and type of new lesions and the response and recurrence of treated lesions. Three months data have been presented at the European Academy of Dermatology and Venereology meeting [19] and show that the number of new lesions in the MAL-PDT treated area is lower than in the area treated with conventional therapy (65 and 103, respectively; $P = .009$). This was mostly related to a decrease in new AK (44 in the MAL-PDT group versus 80 in the conventional therapy group) because the number of new warts did not differ significantly between the two groups (21 and 23).

Prevention of basal cell carcinoma

Oseroff and colleagues [20] described two cases of children with Gorlin's syndrome and multiple BCCs that were treated with large surface ALA-PDT under general anesthesia. One of these children had received radiotherapy in the past to treat meduloblastoma. They reported an excellent response and no recurrence in the treated area with a follow-up of up to 6 years. They also observed that not only BCCs responded to ALA-PDT in these patients but also follicular hamartoma.

Itkin and Gilchrest [21] treated two cases of Gorlin's syndrome with large surface ALA-PDT (two sessions, 1 week apart, repeated after 2 or 4 months). They did not see new BCC lesions in the PDT-treated areas during 8 months of follow-up. Chapas and Gilchrest [22] also reported the case of a 73-year-old patient with Gorlin's syndrome with multiple BCCs on the face that they treated with full-face ALA-PDT for a total of four sessions administered every 2 to 3 months. Blu-U exposure took place 1 hour after ALA application. They noted a significant improvement in the size and number of existing BCCs. They did not mention if there was a decrease in new lesions.

Mechanism of action of skin cancer prevention by photodynamic therapy

The mechanisms involved in the prevention of skin cancer by ALA and MAL-PDT are currently unknown. Experiments conducted with hairless mice where MAL-PDT was applied on one half of the body and vehicle PDT on the other half suggest that the mechanism is mostly local rather than systemic because a delay in skin cancer appearance was only observed on the side where MAL-PDT was performed [11].

In vitro and in vivo studies have shown that there is preferential buildup of porphyrins in neoplastic cells as compared with normal cells [23–25], possibly because of decreased ferrochelatase activity, which converts protoporphyrin IX into heme [26]. A simple potential explanation for the delay in skin cancer appearance observed with PDT is that multiple ALA-PDT or MAL-PDT sessions destroy microscopic foci of AKs before they are clinically visible. To explore this possibility we used the hairless mouse model to study the histologic localization of photodamage following ALA-PDT and the localization of clusters of cells harboring mutations in the p53 gene. ALA-PDT conditions used were similar to experimental conditions that induced a delay in skin cancer appearance. Clusters of cells with mutated p53 have been identified in the epidermis of mice exposed chronically to UV radiation and in patients with extensive sun exposure [27]. These areas are believed to correspond to precursors of AK. In these studies clusters of mutated p53 cells were located in the lower portion of the epidermis, whereas photodamaged cells after ALA-PDT were always located in the upper portion of the epidermis (unpublished data). These studies suggest that, at least in the hairless mouse model, the delay in skin cancer appearance is not caused by a direct phototoxic reaction in clusters of keratinocytes harboring mutations in the p53 gene.

PDT is a complex modality that has been shown to induce the production of cytokines and the induction of tumor-specific immunity in animal models [28–30]. It is possible that some of these phenomena are involved in the delay in skin cancer appearance observed with multiple ALA-PDT sessions.

Summary

Results from preclinical and clinical studies suggest that large surface MAL-PDT and ALA-PDT could prevent the appearance of AK and skin cancer. For patients with lesions on trunk and limbs the efficacy of this approach in clearing existing lesions seems to be enhanced with prior curettage of AK. The best waveband, photosensitizer, time between MAL or ALA application and light exposure, and the best fluence to prevent the development of AK and SCCs have yet to be determined. One of the most important factors determining the success of skin cancer prevention with large surface PDT is treatment frequency. At the current time the best PDT treatment regimen to prevent AK and skin cancer is unknown and it is possible that the optimal treatment regiment will be different for immunosuppressed and immunocompetent patients.

References

[1] Hamzavi I, Lui H. Using light in dermatology: an update on lasers, ultraviolet phototherapy, and photodynamic therapy. Dermatol Clin 2005;23:199–207.

[2] Fukuda H, Casas A, Batlle A. Aminolevulinic acid: from its unique biological function to its star role in photodynamic therapy. Int J Biochem Cell Biol 2005;37:272–6.

[3] de Gruijl FR, Forbes PD. UV-induced skin cancer in a hairless mouse model. Bioessays 1995;17:651–60.

[4] de Gruijl FR, van der Leun JC. Development of skin tumours in hairless mice after discontinuation of ultraviolet irradiation. Cancer Res 1991;51:979–84.

[5] Stender IM, Beck-Thomsen N, Poulsen T, et al. Photodynamic therapy with topical delta-aminolevulinic acid delays UV photocardinogenesis in hairless mice. Photochem Photobiol 1997;66:493–6.

[6] Sharfaei S, Viau G, Lui H, et al. Systemic photodynamic therapy with aminolevulinic acid delays the appearance of ultraviolet-induced skin tumours in mice. Br J Dermatol 2001;144:1207–14.

[7] Liu Y, Viau G, Bissonnette R. Multiple large-surface photodynamic therapy sessions with topical or systemic aminolevulinic acid and blue light in UV-Exposed hairless mice. J Cutan Med Surg 2004;8:131–9.

[8] Bissonnette R, Bergeron A, Liu Y. Large surface photodynamic therapy with aminolevulinic acid: treatment of actinic keratoses and beyond. J Drugs Dermatol 2004;3:S26–31.

[9] Gibbs NK, Young AR, Magnus IA. A strain of hairless mouse susceptible to tumorigenesis by TPA alone: studies with 8-methoxypsoralen and solar simulated radiation. Carcinogenesis 1985;6:797–9.

[10] Juzenas P, Sharfaei S, Moan J, et al. Protoporphyrin IX fluorescence kinetics in UV-induced tumours and normal skin of hairless mice after topical application of 5-aminolevulinic acid methyl ester. J Photochem Photobiol B 2002;67:11–7.

[11] Sharfaei S, Juzenas P, Moan J, et al. Weekly topical application of methyl aminolevulinate followed by light exposure delays the appearance of UV-induced skin tumours in mice. Arch Dermatol Res 2002;294:237–42.

[12] Saldanha G, Fletcher A, Slater DN. Basal cell carcinoma: a dermatopathological and molecular biological update. Br J Dermatol 2003;148:195–202.

[13] Caty V, Liu Y, Viau G, et al. Multiple large surface photodynamic therapy sessions with topical methyl-aminolevulinate in *PTCH* heterozygous mice. Br J Dermatol 2006;154:740–2.

[14] Aszterbaum M, Epstein J, Oro A, et al. Ultraviolet and ionizing radiation enhance the growth of BCCs and trichoblastomas in patched heterozygous knockout mice. Nat Med 1999;5:1285–91.

[15] Wulf HC, Pavel S, Stender IM, et al. Topical photodynamic therapy for prevention of new skin lesions in renal transplant recipients. Presented at the 13th Congress of the European Academy of Dermatology and Venereology (EADV), Florence, Italy, November 18–24, 2004.

[16] de Graaf YG, Kennedy C, Wolterbeek R, et al. Photodynamic therapy does not prevent cutaneous squamous-cell carcinoma in organ-transplant recipients: results of a randomized-controlled trial. J Invest Dermatol 2006;126:569–74.

[17] Dragieva G, Prinz BM, Hafner J, et al. A randomized controlled clinical trial of topical photodynamic therapy with methyl aminolaevulinate in the treatment of actinic keratoses in transplant recipients. Br J Dermatol 2004;151:196–200.

[18] Oseroff A. PDT as a cytotoxic agent and biological response modifier: implications for cancer prevention and treatment in immunosuppressed and immunocompetent patients. J Invest Dermatol 2006;126: 542–4.

[19] Wennberg AM, Keohane S, Lear JT. A multicenter study with MAL-PDT cream in immuno-compromised organ transplant recipients with non-melanoma skin cancer. Poster presented at the European Academy of Dermatology and Venereology (EADV) meeting, London, October 13–16, 2005.

[20] Oseroff AR, Shieh S, Frawley NP, et al. Treatment of diffuse basal cell carcinomas and basaloid follicular hamartomas in nevoid basal cell carcinoma syndrome by wide-area 5-aminolevulinic acid photodynamic therapy. Arch Dermatol 2005;141:60–7.

[21] Itkin A, Gilchrest BA. delta-Aminolevulinic acid and blue light photodynamic therapy for treatment of multiple basal cell carcinomas in two patients with nevoid basal cell carcinoma syndrome. Dermatol Surg 2004;30:1054–61.

[22] Chapas AM, Gilchrest BA. Broad area photodynamic therapy for treatment of multiple basal cell carcinomas in a patient with nevoid basal cell carcinoma syndrome. J Drugs Dermatol 2006;5(2 Suppl): 3–5.

[23] Angell-Petersen E, Sorensen R, Warloe T, et al. Porphyrin formation in actinic keratosis and basal cell carcinoma after topical application of methyl 5-aminolevulinate. J Invest Dermatol 2006;126:265–71.

[24] Fritsch C, Homey B, Stahl W, et al. Preferential relative porphyrin enrichment in solar keratoses upon topical application of aminolevulinic acid methylester. Photochem Photobiol 1998;68:218–21.

[25] Peng QA, Warloe T, Moan J, et al. Distribution of 5-aminolevulinic acid-induced porphyrins in noduloulcerative basal cell carcinoma. Photochem Photobiol 1995;62:906–13.

[26] Rittenhouse-Diakun K, Van Leengoed H, Morgan J, et al. The role of transferrin receptor (CD71) in photodynamic therapy of activated and malignant lymphocytes using the heme precursor delta-aminolevulinic acid (ALA). Photochem Photobiol 1995;61: 523–8.

[27] Berg JWR, van Kranen HJ, Rebel HG. Early p53 alterations in mouse skin carcinogenesis by UVB radiation: immunohistochemical detection of mutant p53 protein in clusters of preneoplastic epidermal cells. Proc Natl Acad Sci U S A 1996;93:274–8.

[28] Canti G, De Simone A, Korbelik M. Photodynamic therapy and the immune system in experimental oncology. Photochem Photobiol Sci 2002;1:79–80.

[29] Gollnick SO, Musser DA, Oseroff AR, et al. IL-10 does not play a role in cutaneous photofrin photodynamic therapy-induced suppression of the contact hypersensitivity response. Photochem Photobiol 2001;74:811–6.

[30] Gollnick SO, Evans SS, Baumann H, et al. Role of cytokines in photodynamic therapy-induced local and systemic inflammation. Br J Cancer 2003;88: 1772–9.

ELSEVIER
SAUNDERS

Dermatol Clin 25 (2007) 101–109

DERMATOLOGIC
CLINICS

Photodynamic Therapy: Other Uses

Amy Forman Taub, MD[a,b,*]

[a]Department of Dermatology, Northwestern University Medical School, Chicago,
676 St. Clair Street, IL 60611, USA
[b]Advanced Dermatology, 275 Parkway Drive, Lincolnshire, IL 60069, USA

Mainstream uses for photodynamic therapy (PDT) in dermatology include nonmelanoma skin cancer and its precursors, acne vulgaris, photo-rejuvenation, and hidradenitis suppurativa. Each one of these entities and more is covered elsewhere in this issue. Many other dermatologic entities have been treated with PDT and published in the literature. These include psoriasis vulgaris, cutaneous T-cell lymphoma (CTCL), disseminated actinic porokeratosis (DSAP), localized scleroderma, and vulval lichen sclerosus (LS). Nondermatologic applications include anal and vulvar carcinoma, palliation of metastatic breast cancer to skin, Barrett's esophagus, and macular degeneration of the retina. These are divided in the following categories and the literature explored in each: nonmelanoma skin cancer, other neoplasia (dermatologic and nondermatologic), inflammatory/immunologic, infectious, and miscellaneous (Table 1).

Nonmelanoma skin cancer

Actinic keratosis, basal cell carcinoma, and squamous cell carcinoma are reviewed elsewhere.

Neither grants nor subsidies were received to prepare this manuscript. The author is a consultant to DUSA pharmaceuticals. Receipt of honoraria for educational activities has been received in the past. The author owns a small amount of stock in DUSA. She also is on the Board of Directors for the American Society for Photodynamic Therapy.

* 275 Parkway Drive, Suite 521, Lincolnshire, IL 60069.

E-mail address: drtaub@skinfo.com

Disseminated superficial actinic porokeratosis

This condition is a clone of actinically damaged cells that have the potential to transform into squamous cell carcinoma; hence, the author chose to put DSAP in this category. The general consensus anecdotally is that PDT is not effective for DSAP; however, only one paper, which treated three patients with topical PDT, is in the literature and the investigators failed to get a response [1]. The author has treated three patients for DSAP with success (unpublished observations). One patient is a 55-year-old woman who had widespread DSAP (legs, arms, back) who had two lesions convert into histologically proven squamous cell carcinoma. She had been treated with imiquimod and 5-flourouracil topically over many years, but developed systemic side effects from both. She has responded well to multiple PDT sessions with 20% aminolevulinic acid (ALA) solution (Levulan, DUSA Pharmaceuticals, Wilmington, Massachusetts). In the author's experience, DSAP can be treated with PDT successfully; however, multiple treatments are necessary at the highest light dosages and longest incubations with some pretreatment of the lesions (5-fluorouracil, imiquimod, salicylic acid containing compounds, retinoids, or a combination thereof). This does clear many of the lesions, which will reoccur over the next 1 to 2 years, and leads to the possibility that annual treatments may be necessary. It is hoped that more case reports and clinical trials will be reported in the future to add to our knowledge of how to treat this difficult disease.

Inflammatory/immunologic disorders

Acne vulgaris and hidradenitis suppurativa are covered elsewhere in this issue.

0733-8635/07/$ - see front matter © 2006 Elsevier Inc. All rights reserved.
doi:10.1016/j.det.2006.09.007

Table 1
Conditions treated by photodynamic therapy

Nonmelanoma skin cancer	Other neoplasia	Inflammatory/immune disorders	Infectious disorders	Miscellaneous
Actinic keratosis[a]	Dermatologic	Acne vulgaris[a]	HPV[a]	Laser-assisted hair removal
Basal cell CA[a]	Cutaneous T-cell lymphoma	Psoriasis	MRSA	
		Lichen planus	Osteomyelitis	
Squamous cell CA[a]	Nondermatologic	Lichen sclerosus	Molluscum contagiosum	
Actinic cheilitis[a]	Vulvar/cervical intraepithelial neoplasia	Scleroderma	Tinea rubrum	
DSAP	Anal carcinoma	Alopecia areata	Oral candidiasis	
	Penile intraepithelial neoplasia	Darier's disease		
	Barrett's esophagus	Hidradenitis suppurativa[a]		
	Breast cancer metastatic to chest wall	Macular degeneration of the retina		

Abbreviations: CA, carcinoma; HPV, human papillomavirus; MRSA, methicillin-resistant *Staphylococcus avreus.*
[a] Not covered in this article; covered in depth in other articles in this issue.

Psoriasis vulgaris

There is a fair amount of literature devoted to the treatment of psoriasis vulgaris with PDT; outcomes are mixed about whether PDT is a practical or useful alternative for treatment.

The first hurdle was to demonstrate the mechanism of action of PDT or preferential uptake of a photosensitizer by psoriatic plaques. Bisonnette and colleagues [2] looked at the potential for specificity of oral ALA in dosages of 10, 20, and 30 mg because they believed that using topical PDT would be too limiting. They measured 12 patients with plaque psoriasis' protoporphyrin IX (PpIX) fluorescence in the lesional and normal skin as well as in inflammatory cells. There was a 10-fold increase in fluorescence at 3 to 5 hours after administration of a single oral dose in the psoriasis over the normal skin, although they did note some fluorescence of noninvolved facial skin. They concluded that this was a modality that warranted potential study for clinical usage. An earlier study [3] had established that PDT with red light caused a similar, although less potent, decrease in cytokine secretions (interleukin [IL]-6, tumor necrosis factor [TNF]-α, IL-1β) as did psoralen plus ultraviolet A light (PUVA) therapy in mononuclear cells that were isolated freshly after irradiation with either modality. It also demonstrated progressive photobleaching corresponding to higher energy irradiations, which established the specificity and dose dependency

for PDT for psoriasis vulgaris. A recent study showed that systemic PDT induces apoptosis in lesional T lymphocytes in psoriatic plaques, a feature that is supposed to predict a longer-lasting therapeutic effect [4].

With some evidence of a mechanistic reason and proof of some specificity for psoriasis vulgaris, small clinical trials were instituted to test whether this was borne out in a clinical setting. Ten patients who had plaque psoriasis [5] were treated multiple times at thrice a week dosing with topical application of 5-ALA and broadband visible radiation at dosage of 8 J/cm^2. Eight out of ten patients showed a clinical response, but only 1 of 45 sites cleared fully and 5 showed no improvement. More concerning was that fluorescence, which was demonstrated by biopsy to remain in the epidermis, showed little consistency of uptake, even within the same plaque. Finally, there was so much discomfort with the treatments that the investigators concluded this was not a practical therapy.

Three studies in 2005 shed new light on the clinical evaluation of PDT for psoriasis vulgaris. Twelve patients (8 evaluable) were studied for their response to topical 5-ALA 20% solution irradiated with red light weekly at 10 to 30 J/cm^2 [6]. There was a statistically significant improvement in the clinical presentation of the plaques; however, there was an average pain score of 7 on the Visual Analogue Scale and 4 of 12 patients dropped out of the study because of pain during the treatments. A larger study was performed by the Regensberg, Germany group; 29 psoriatics who had chronic stable disease received 1% ALA after keratolytic treatment (10% salicylic acid in petrolatum for 2 weeks) in three plaques and 5, 10, or 20 J/cm^2 of a filtered metal halide light (Waldmann 1200 PDT, 600–740 nm) [7]. Although they demonstrated a clear decrease in the psoriasis severity area index score in more than 95% of patients, the slow pace, pain during therapy, and partial results were cited by the investigators as reasons for the inadequacy of this form of PDT for psoriasis vulgaris. They concluded that a more practical method might be oral ALA and blue light or verteporfin and red light. Finally, in a recent study, 8 patients who had symmetric plaques were studied for clinical response and immunohistochemical markers in a randomized, placebo-controlled study in which the patient's contralateral plaque served as control [8]. Ten percent ALA ointment under occlusion was used on one plaque, whereas the vehicle alone was used on the contralateral plaque; both were occluded for 4 hours and exposed to fractionated broadband light (Waldmann PDT 1200 L, 650–700 nm) at 2 J/cm^2, then 2 dark hours, followed by 8 J/cm^2. The PDT-treated side exhibited a clinical improvement and a decrease in CD4$^+$, CD8$^+$, and CD450RO cells as well as Ki67$^+$ nuclei, with an increase in epidermal K10 expression. These biologic changes were absent in the placebo-treated sides. Heterogeneity of plaques in fluorescent staining still was seen as an obstacle to practical therapy, and this was despite pretreatment with a salicylic acid–based cream to induce keratolysis. Still, despite a modest clinical result, the investigators hold out hope that protocols could be optimized for psoriatic therapy.

Psoriasis treatment for PDT seems to be limited by pain, inconvenience, and mediocre results. Clearly, it is not a first-line therapy; however, there is good evidence that there is preferential uptake of photosensitizers in psoriatic plaques and confirmation by biologic markers that specific antipsoriatic changes take place during PDT. Therefore, it is hoped that there will be a way to optimize PDT protocols for the treatment of psoriasis.

Lichen planus

There is only one reference, a recent study in the use of PDT, for the treatment of oral lichen planus (OLP). Twenty-six lesions of OLP were treated with gargling 5% methylene blue and subsequent irradiation with 632-nm laser at 120 J/cm^2. Significant symptoms and signs were decreased at 1 and 12 weeks in 16 lesions; the investigators concluded that this was a promising treatment for control of OLP [9].

Lichen sclerosus

This entity is mentioned twice in overviews of PDT and once by Polish investigators who stated they use PDT for diagnosis and treatment of LS; however, the full text could not be obtained and there were no details in the abstract [10].

Scleroderma

Patients who had localized scleroderma that was resistant to PUVA did respond well to PDT [11]. Cultured keratinocytes that were subjected to PDT produced increased IL-1, TNF, and matrix metallopreoteinase-1 and -3; these were postulated by the investigators to be the mechanisms that are responsible for the observed antisclerotic effect of PDT [12]. This observation needs to be repeated and is contrary to what is found clinically with photodynamic photorejuvenation (ie, fine wrinkles tend to get better and there has been no evidence of collagen breakdown). Another study, however, found a dosimetry range to reduce tissue contraction and reduce collagen density without damage to keratinocytes, which may prove helpful as an adjuvant treatment for keloids [13].

Alopecia areata

Six patients who had severe alopecia areata were treated with 5% to 15% ALA solution twice weekly for 20 treatments with red light. Fluorescence microscopy revealed diffuse uptake in the epidermis and sebaceous glands, but not in hair follicles or the inflammatory infiltrate surrounding the epidermis. Also, a significant degree of erythema was noted in all ALA-treated sites but not in the control site, which indicated that there was a clinical response to ALA. The investigators concluded that PDT is not a successful therapy for alopecia areata [14].

Darier's disease

A small pilot study of six patients was treated with 5-ALA; they also were taking systemic retinoids. One patient could not tolerate treatment. Of the other five patients, four had an inflammatory response that lasted for 2 weeks, but it was followed by improvement that lasted from 6 to 36 months. There was recurrence in one patient; however, in those who were clear, biopsy was negative after treatment [15].

Macular degeneration of the retina

Macular degeneration of the retina occurs as an age-related phenomenon when new vessels under the retina proliferate and leak, which causes distortion and scarring and leads to reduction of visual acuity, and, ultimately, blindness. Use of PDT for this condition has made a previously untreatable disease treatable. Verteporfin is used as the photosensitizer; it is followed by a series of three to six treatments over 1 to 2 years, which results in a decrease of loss of vision relative to untreated controls, and, in some instances, an improvement of vision. This was approved by the US Food and Drug Administration in 2000 and has been used in more than 1 million applications [16].

The mechanism of action is induction of apoptosis in the endothelial cells in the proliferating vessels, which is specific and leaves the rest of the retina intact [17]. Investigators in this area disagree on whether PDT is appropriate in late-stage disease. In one study, 8 of 10 patients lost less than three lines of vision over 2 years in late disease [18]; however, in another study, many of the patients who had advanced disease had significant side effects after usage [19]. A Cochrane analysis of the literature concluded that PDT is safe and effective for treatment of macular degeneration of the retina, although the size of the effect is not understood completely [20]. There is a newer alternative therapy that involved injection of the drug anecortave acetate. In a recent comparative study this was shown to be about as effective as PDT [21].

Other neoplasia: dermatologic

Cutaneous T-cell lymphoma

Traditionally, treatment of early CTCL has been accomplished with PUVA, electron beam radiation, nitrogen mustard, and even topical steroids. It seems a logical consequence that PDT might be effective for CTCL because it is effective in other neoplasias of skin. Many pilot studies and cases report positive findings, although no large-scale studies have been reported. The first reported treatment of CTCL was in 1994, when two plaque lesions were treated with 20%

ALA in water-in-oil–based cream, and incubation for 4 to 6 hours followed by laser irradiation [22]. PpIX production was demonstrated by real-time laser-induced fluorescence to have a fivefold increase in lymphoma cells over normal cells. In 1995, Oseroff's group hypothesized that activated lymphocytes (CD71$^+$) would accumulate PpIX preferentially because of their lower intracellular iron levels and because of competition for iron between ALA-induced heme production and cellular growth processes [23]. They demonstrated that incubation of ALA with the CD71 positive lymphocytes from a patient with Sezary syndrome was killed preferentially over normal, unstimulated lymphocytes, which indicated a possible mechanism for PDT as well as specificity for CTCL and potential for good clinical outcomes.

In 1999, Eich and colleagues [24] reported two cases, one of an uncommon type and location of CTCL (medium-large size pleiomorphic cells, CD8$^+$, CD30$^-$, ear) that had not responded to PUVA, interferon-α, or retinoid therapy, but achieved a histologically confirmed partial remission with PDT and subsequent complete remission (CR) with radiotherapy. A second patient had PDT to the eyebrow and the foot in combination with other modalities to effect a CR. In 2000, Orenstein and colleagues [25] presented two patients who had stages I and III CTCL. In stage I CTCL, lesions exhausted fluorescence 1 hour after irradiation and showed a good response with 170 J/cm^2. With the stage III lesion, fractionated dosages were necessary, with a total dose required of 380 J/cm^2. All six lesions responded well. Other case reports include successful treatment of a patient who had two isolated plaques [26] and a patient infected with HIV who had CTCL and achieved CR after two PDT treatment cycles [27].

In the largest study to date, Ros' group in Sweden examined 10 patients with 10 plaque and 2 tumor-stage lesions [28]. They also looked at histologic and immunohistochemical markers of the lesions. The protocol was 20% ALA, incubating for 6 hours, followed with red light. Complete clinical remission was noted in 7 of 10 plaques after a single treatment, with corresponding regression of infiltrate with markedly fewer proliferating cells and a decrease in Ki-67 and CD71. The tumor lesions did not respond. The investigators concluded that there was good clinical and histologic effect of PDT on local plaque CTCL.

In summary, the literature demonstrates a good response to PDT for localized plaque

CTCL, stage I in case reports and limited pilot studies, which were confirmed clinically, histologically, and by way of immunohistochemistry. A plausible mechanism for action and specificity has been postulated and demonstrated partially. Further large-scale studies are necessary to evaluate whether PDT will be useful in treating early CTCL, but it certainly would be warranted if other modalities had failed or if circumstances preclude patients from receiving other, more established, modalities.

Other neoplasia: nondermatologic

Any epithelial cancer or precursor lesion that is accessible to light irradiation can be treated with PDT. Mucous membranes are especially well-suited to PDT because of the increased permeability in the absence of a well-developed stratum corneum. Thus, vulvar, cervical, and anal carcinomas have been treated by PDT with some success.

Vulvar intraepithelial neoplasia

Vulvar intraepithelial neoplasia (VIN) grades I–III was treated with 20% solution of 5-ALA and treated with 100 J/cm^2 of laser light at 635 nm in 25 patients who had 111 lesions. Complete response was noted in 13 patients (52% who had 27 lesions. All patients who had VIN grade I and monofocal or bifocal VIN grades II–III showed complete clearance. Multifocal VIN grades II–III lesions were cleared only 27% of the time. The investigators concluded that PDT was a good alternative for VIN grades I–III uni- or bifocal disease, whereas multifocal, pigmented, and hyperkeratotic lesions were not amenable to clearance. Advantages of PDT include excellent cosmesis and function with minimal morbidity; disadvantages include the need for close surveillance of recurrence [29].

In another study, 22 patients who had VIN grades II–III had 10% 5-ALA applied for 2 to 4 hours and 80 to 125 J/cm^2 light at 635 nm. This was compared with CO_2 laser and surgical excision for VIN grade III. The complete response rate for VIN proven by biopsy was 57%. Reduced disease-free survival was related to multifocal lesions, regardless of therapy type. PDT was concluded to be as effective as conventional therapy, but it had shorter healing times and better cosmetic results [30].

A different photosensitizer, meta-tetrahydroxyphenylchlorin, in VIN grade III was injected intravenously (IV) at 0.1 mg/kg body weight and irradiated 96 hours later with a 652-nm diode laser. Patients healed without incident except for two cases of severe pain that lasted for 2 weeks and one case of cellulitis. At 6 months, two patients developed recurrence and one had a new site; all were retreated with PDT. At 2 years, there were no recurrences at the original site, and cosmesis and functional anatomy were preserved well [31].

Cervical intraepithelial neoplasia

Similar findings, albeit with less confirmatory studies, exist for cervical neoplasia and PDT. A recent comparison of PDT plus topical 5-ALA with cold-knife conization yielded similar clearance rates (75%) of human papillomavirus (HPV) at 3 months and disease-free rates at 12 months (PDT, 91%; cold-knife, 100%). PDT preserved the function and structure of the cervix better than did surgery; however, the investigators warned that close long-term follow-up is warranted [32]. Another study of 3% ALA in gel incubated for 3 hours with loop excision performed 3 months after PDT in 12 patients found no significant difference between PDT and placebo [33].

In a larger and more recent study, 105 patients who had CIN received Photofrin, 2 mg/kg IV, and were treated with a laser at 630 nm at 100 J/cm^2. CR was 90% at 3 months and 72% at 12 months, with eradication of HPV in 75%. Three patients required surgery 2 to 4 years after the PDT. The investigators concluded that this is an effective method for the treatment of CIN [34].

Penile intraepithelial neoplasia

Penile intraepithelial neoplasia (PIN) is difficult to treat and can require mutilating surgery. Ten patients who had PIN were treated with PDT. Two of 10 patients were cured with four or five treatments. Patients required a penile block to be able to tolerate the pain of the procedure; 50% of them had concurrent HPV-16, whereas 30% had LS. None of the patients was circumcised. The investigators concluded that prevention (circumcision) is better than treatment; however, even with only a 20% response rate this may be an alternative to mutilating surgery [35].

Anal carcinoma in situ

Anal carcinoma in situ is another mucosal surface cancer that is accessible to PDT. Twelve patients who had active HIV and high-grade dysplasia of anal mucosa were given oral δ-ALA and light irradiation. All patients had a downgrading of dysplasia on follow-up at 5 months as measured by Papanicolaou smears. The investigators conclude that this is a useful treatment alternative to surgery in anal carcinoma in situ [36]. In another study, 13 patients were treated with oral ALA and IV Photofrin with a 633-nm diode laser treatment. Patients required 2 days of anesthesia and no sun, 2 weeks of hospitalization, and 8 weeks to recover. Eight of 13 patients had a complete response and were able to avoid disfiguring surgery [37].

In conclusion, CIN and VIN seem to be treated well with PDT if the lesions are not multifocal, pigmented, or hyperkeratotic as long as rigorous long-term follow-up is maintained and biopsies do not demonstrate invasive cancer. In addition, cosmesis and function are better preserved with PDT than with surgical treatments or destructions. Penile and anal carcinomas are much more difficult to eradicate; the treatments have long recoveries and are extremely painful with results that are not as good, but they may be warranted because the alternatives are mutilating surgeries.

Barrett's esophagus

The treatment of Barrett's esophagus, a precancerous/in situ lesion of the epithelial lining, had been on two extreme sides: periodic endoscopy with focal resections or total esophagectomy. PDT has become an important alternative, with varying degrees of success for low-grade and high-grade dysplasia. Twenty-six men who had mainly low-grade dysplasia were randomized to receive focal ablation with an argon plasma coagulator or PDT with IV Photofrin and 630-nm laser. PDT performed superiorly in eradicating dysplasia, although both were able to shorten the duration of the lesions [38]. A recent long-term study demonstrated that 20 men who had high-grade dysplasia of the esophagus had good response to PDT [39]. A dose-response study demonstrated that higher-dose light resulted in better ablation of lesions, but with more complications (eg, stricture, esophagitis) [40].

Breast cancer metastatic to chest wall

Palliation of pain and reducing difficult wound care are the goals of treating breast cancer that is metastatic to chest wall, which occurs in 5% of patients who have breast cancer. Eighteen patients with more than 500 truncal metastases were treated with IV Photofrin and 630-nm diode laser. Follow-up was from 6 to 24 months, with 9 of 14 complete responses; some tumors that were greater than 2-cm thick responded. The investigators concluded that this is a worthwhile treatment for palliation with excellent clinical response [41].

Infectious disorders

There is evidence that PDT can be active against bacteria, viruses, and fungi.

Bacteria

In 1990, it was demonstrated that *Escherichia coli* could be killed if pretreated with methylene blue and exposed to white light [42]. *Helicobacter* infection was eradicated with methylene and toluidine blue, using a copper vapor–pumped dye laser on ex vivo samples of ferret gastric mucosa, without damage to the underlying mucosa [43]. A novel porphyrin-based photosensitizer, XF73, showed high efficacy at killing methicillin-resistant *Staphylococcus aureus* (MRSA) without damage to keratinocytes or eukaryotic cells [44]. The investigators postulated a use for this photosensitizer to prevent MRSA infection in hospitals as well as for burns or other open wounds [45]. Mice that were infected with bacteria were saved from sepsis and had improved wound healing after PDT [46]. In other mouse studies, third-degree burns were treated with PDT; 98% of the bacteria were eradicated after one session [47]. Fifty-three percent of 19 mice that were infected with *Vibrio vulnificus* at a bacterial inoculation 100 times the lethal dose for 50% survived after being treated with 100 μg of toluene blue and red light (150 J/cm^2) [48]. *Staphylococcus aureus*–infected mouse bone was treated with PDT successfully [49]. This in vivo animal model was used to postulate that PDT might be a good therapeutic alternative for the treatment of osteomyelitis.

Fungi

PDT was shown to have in vitro effects against *Tinea rubrum* at dosages of ALA of 1 to 10 mmol and 10 to 14 days of incubation [50]. Diode laser was effective in activating toluene blue–induced PDT of *Candida* species at low levels [51]. Mice that had severe combined immunodeficiency developed mucocutaneous candidiasis that was treated successfully with methylene blue and 664-nm diode laser in a dose-dependent fashion. This led the investigators to conclude that this could be a viable treatment options for humans [52]. Interdigital tinea pedis was treated successfully with 29% ALA in Eucerin cream and 75 J/cm^2 red light. The control group (light alone or ALA alone) had no response; however, four of nine patients had recurrence of disease within 4 weeks of therapy [53].

Viruses

The most literature on viral diseases that are treated with PDT regards warts or condylomata (also see elsewhere in this issue). Other viruses that were reported to be treated with PDT include molluscum contagiosum [54] and herpes simplex [55,56]. Other uses of PDT include inactivating pathogens from blood products before infusion [57].

In summary, PDT was shown in vitro and in animal models to be highly effective for various pathogens, including MRSA and candidiasis, in immunocompromised hosts. The varied organisms that were tested do not seem to be capable of mounting a defense or developing resistant strains to PDT. In addition, photosensitizers continue to be discovered that are specific to the pathogenic targets and are not mutagenic. Localized skin infections, chronic wounds, or oral candidiasis probably is the most convenient targets for PDT [57]. PDT shows great promise as a weapon against MRSA and other pathogens that easily develop resistance. This promise begs more research to transform PDT for anti-infective use from the exploratory phase to a clinical reality.

Miscellaneous

Hair removal

PDT was performed with ALA after cold wax epilation and a continuous-wave red laser. Hair removal was consistent with the amount of anagen hair present [58]. Alopecia presented as a side effect in a case report of treatment of Bowen's disease with 5-ALA and red laser light on an upper posterior arm. The tumor was eradicated after 2-years follow-up, but complete alopecia of the treatment area remained [59]. There are few data to support the use of PDT as an adjunct to laser hair removal, and there have been few reports of alopecia as a side effect of treatments. There has been no demonstration of specific uptake by hair follicle cells. The author has not found PDT useful anecdotally as an adjuvant for laser-assisted hair removal.

Overview of other uses of photodynamic therapy

PDT is useful in nonmelanoma skin cancers, immunologic and inflammatory disorders, neoplasias other than skin cancer, and infections. The ability of this treatment to hone in on dysplastic epithelial and endothelial cells while retaining viability of surrounding tissue is its key feature, because this leads to specific tumor destruction with cosmesis and function of the target organ intact. The ability of PDT to alter the course of immunologic and inflammatory diseases is in an exploratory stage, but one that is exciting to behold and certainly is well established for diseases of sebaceous glands, and, possibly, apocrine glands. Finally, the demonstration that PDT is capable of killing various pathogens without induction of resistance could make it an important treatment modality in this arena in the future.

References

[1] Nayeemuddin FA, Wong M, Yell J, et al. Topical photodynamic therapy in disseminated superficial actinic porokeratosis. Clin Exp Dermatol 2002; 27(8):703–6.

[2] Bissonnette R, Zeng H, McLean DI, et al. Oral aminolevulinic acid induces protoporphyrin IX fluorescence in psoriatic plaques and peripheral blood cells. Photochem Photobiol 2001;74(2):339–45.

[3] Boehncke WH, Konig K, Kaufmann R, et al. Photodynamic therapy in psoriasis: suppression of cytokine production in vitro and recording of fluorescence modification during treatment in vivo. Arch Dermatol Res 1994;286(6):300–3.

[4] Bissonnette R, Tremblay JF, Juzenas P, et al. Systemic photodynamic therapy with aminolevulinic acid induces apoptosis in lesional T lymphocytes of psoriatic plaques. J Invest Dermatol 2002;119(1): 77–83.

[5] Robinson DJ, Collins P, Stringer MR, et al. Improved response of plaque psoriasis after multiple treatments with topical 5-aminolaevulinic acid photodynamic therapy. Acta Derm Venereol 1999;79(6): 451–5.

[6] Fransson J, Ros AM. Clinical and immunohistochemical evaluation of psoriatic plaques treated with topical 5-aminolaevulinic acid photodynamic therapy. Photodermatol Photoimmunol Photomed 2005;21(6):326–32.

[7] Radakovic-Fijan S, Blecha-Thalhammer U, Schleyer V, et al. Topical aminolaevulinic acid–based photodynamic therapy as a treatment option for psoriasis? Results of a randomized, observer-blinded study. Br J Dermatol 2005;152(2): 279–83.

[8] Smits T, Kleinpenning MM, van Erp PEJ, et al. A placebo-controlled randomized study on the clinical effectiveness, immunohistochemical changes and protoporphyrin IX accumulation in fractionated 5-aminolaevulinic acid-photodynamic therapy in patients with psoriasis. Br J Dermatol 2006;155(3): 539–45.

[9] Aghahosseini F, Arbabi-Kalati F, Fashtami LA, et al. Methylene blue-mediated photodynamic therapy: a possible alternative treatment for oral lichen planus. Lasers Surg Med 2006;38(1):33–8.

[10] Olejek A, Rembielak-Stawecka B, Kozak-Darmas I, et al. Photodynamic diagnosis and therapy in gynecology–current knowledge [in Polish]. Ginekol Pol 2004;75(3):228–34.

[11] Szeimies RM, Landthaler M, Karrer S. Non-oncologic indications for ALA-PDT. J Dermatolog Treat 2002;13(Suppl 1):S13–8.

[12] Karrer S, Bosserhoff AK, Weiderer P, et al. Keratinocyte-derived cytokines after photodynamic therapy and their paracrine induction of matrix metalloproteinases in fibroblasts. Br J Dermatol 2004;151(4):776–83.

[13] Chiu LL, Sun CH, Yeh AT, et al. Photodynamic therapy on keloid fibroblasts in tissue-engineered keratinocyte-fibroblast co-culture. Lasers Surg Med 2005;37(3):231–44.

[14] Bissonnette R, Shapiro J, Zeng H, et al. Topical photodynamic therapy with 5-aminolaevulinic acid does not induce hair regrowth in patients with extensive alopecia areata. Br J Dermatol 2000;143(5): 1032–5.

[15] Exadaktylou D, Kurwa HA, Calonje E, et al. Treatment of Darier's disease with photodynamic therapy. Br J Dermatol 2003;149(3):606–10.

[16] Wickens J, Blinder KJ. A preliminary benefit-risk assessment of verteporfin in age-related macular degeneration. Drug Saf 2006;29(3):189–99.

[17] Potter MJ, Szabo SM. Verteporfin photodynamic therapy–induced apoptosis in choroidal neovascular membranes. Br J Ophthalmol 2006; [epub ahead of print].

[18] Petermeier K, Tatar O, Inhoffen W, et al. One-year outcomes after photodynamic therapy in patients with age-related macular degeneration with poor baseline visual acuity. Graefes Arch Clin Exp Ophthalmol 2005;1–3.

[19] Boscia F, Parodi MB, Furino C, et al. Photodynamic therapy with verteporfin for retinal angiomatous proliferation. Graefes Arch Clin Exp Ophthalmol 2006;244(10):1224–32.

[20] Wormald R, Evans J, Smeeth L, et al. Photodynamic therapy for neovascular age-related macular degeneration. Cochrane Database Syst Rev 2005;(4): CD002030.

[21] Slakter JS, Bochow TW, D'Amico DJ, et al. Anecortave Acetate Clinical Study Group. Anecortave acetate (15 milligrams) versus photodynamic therapy for treatment of subfoveal neovascularization in age-related macular degeneration. Ophthalmology 2006;113(1):3–13.

[22] Svanberg K, Andersson T, Killander D, et al. Photodynamic therapy of non-melanoma malignant tumours of the skin using topical delta-amino levulinic acid sensitization and laser irradiation. Br J Dermatol 1994;130(6):743–51.

[23] Rittenhouse-Diakun K, Van Leengoed H, Morgan J, et al. The role of transferrin receptor (CD71) in photodynamic therapy of activated and malignant lymphocytes using the heme precursor delta-amino-levulinic acid (ALA). Photochem Photobiol 1995; 61(5):523–8.

[24] Eich D, Eich HT, Otte HG, et al. Photodynamic therapy of cutaneous T-cell lymphoma at special sites [in German]. Hautarzt 1999;50(2):109–14.

[25] Orenstein A, Haik J, Tamir J, et al. Photodynamic therapy of cutaneous lymphoma using 5-aminolevulinic acid topical application. Dermatol Surg 2000; 26(8):765–9 [discussion 769–70].

[26] Leman JA, Dick DC, Morton CA. Topical 5-ALA photodynamic therapy for the treatment of cutaneous T-cell lymphoma. Clin Exp Dermatol 2002; 27(6):516–8.

[27] Paech V, Lorenzen T, Stoehr A, et al. Remission of cutaneous Mycosis fungoides after topical 5-ALA sensitization and photodynamic therapy in a patient with advanced HIV-infection. Eur J Med Res 2002; 7(11):477–9.

[28] Edstrom DW, Porwit A, Ros AM. Photodynamic therapy with topical 5-aminolevulinic acid for Mycosis fungoides: clinical and histological response. Acta Derm Venereol 2001;81(3):184–8.

[29] Hillemanns P, Untch M, Dannecker C, et al. Photodynamic therapy of vulvar intraepithelial neoplasia using 5-aminolevulinic acid. Int J Cancer 2000; 85(5):649–53.

[30] Fehr MK, Hornung R, Degen A, et al. Photodynamic therapy of vulvar and vaginal condyloma and intraepithelial neoplasia using topically applied 5-aminolevulinic acid. Lasers Surg Med 2002;30(4): 273–9.

[31] Campbell SM, Gould DJ, Salter L, et al. Photodynamic therapy using meta-tetrahydroxyphenyl-chlorin (Foscan) for the treatment of vulval intraepithelial neoplasia. Br J Dermatol 2004; 151(5):1076–80.

[32] Bodner K, Bodner-Adler B, Wierrani F, et al. Cold-knife conization versus photodynamic therapy with topical 5-aminolevulinic acid (5-ALA) in cervical intraepithelial neoplasia (CIN) II with associated human papillomavirus infection: a comparison of preliminary results. Anticancer Res 2003;23(2C): 1785–8.

[33] Barnett AA, Haller JC, Cairnduff F, et al. A randomised, double-blind, placebo-controlled trial of photodynamic therapy using 5-aminolaevulinic acid for the treatment of cervical intraepithelial neoplasia. Int J Cancer 2003;103(6):829–32.

[34] Yamaguchi S, Tsuda H, Takemori M, et al. Photodynamic therapy for cervical intraepithelial neoplasia. Oncology 2005;69(2):110–6.

[35] Wennberg AM. Our experience with penile intraepithelias neoplasia. Presented at the Euro-PDT Annual Meeting. Bern, Switzerland, March 31–April 1, 2006.

[36] Webber J, Fromm D. Photodynamic therapy for carcinoma in situ of the anus. Arch Surg 2004; 139(3):259–61.

[37] Warloe T. PDT for anal cancer in situ. Presented at the Euro-PDT 2006 Annual Meeting. Bern, Switzerland, March 31–April 1, 2006.

[38] Ragunath K, Krasner N, Raman VS, et al. Endoscopic ablation of dysplastic Barrett's oesophagus comparing argon plasma coagulation and photodynamic therapy: a randomized prospective trial assessing efficacy and cost-effectiveness. Scand J Gastroenterol 2005;40(7):750–8.

[39] Foroulis CN, Thorpe JA. Photodynamic therapy (PDT) in Barrett's esophagus with dysplasia or early cancer. Eur J Cardiothorac Surg 2006;29(1):30–4.

[40] Kelty CJ, Ackroyd R, Brown NJ, et al. Comparison of high- vs low-dose 5-aminolevulinic acid for photodynamic therapy of Barrett's esophagus. Surg Endosc 2004;18(3):452–8.

[41] Cuenca RE, Allison RR, Sibata C, et al. Breast cancer with chest wall progression: treatment with photodynamic therapy. Ann Surg Oncol 2004; 11(3):332–7.

[42] Menezes S, Capella MA, Caldas LR. Photodynamic action of methylene blue: repair and mutation in *Escherichia coli.* J Photochem Photobiol B 1990; 5(3–4):505–17.

[43] Millson CE, Wilson M, MacRobert AJ, et al. Ex-vivo treatment of gastric *Helicobacter* infection by photodynamic therapy. J Photochem Photobiol B 1996;32(1–2):59–65.

[44] Maisch T, Bosl C, Szeimies RM, et al. Photodynamic effects of novel XF porphyrin derivatives on prokaryotic and eukaryotic cells. Antimicrob Agents Chemother 2005;49(4):1542–52.

[45] Maisch T. Phototoxicity of a novel porphyrin photosensitizer against MRSA in an ex-vivo porcine skin model. Presented at the Sixth annual Euro-PDT Meeting. Berne, Switzerland, March 31–April 1, 2006.

[46] Demidova TN, Hamblin MR. Photodynamic therapy targeted to pathogens. Int J Immunopathol Pharmacol 2004;17(3):245–54.

[47] Lambrechts SA, Demidova TN, Aalders MC, et al. Photodynamic therapy for *Staphylococcus aureus* infected burn wounds in mice. Photochem Photobiol Sci 2005;4(7):503–9.

[48] Wong TW, Wang YY, Sheu HM, et al. Bactericidal effects of toluidine blue–mediated photodynamic action on *Vibrio vulnificus.* Antimicrob Agents Chemother 2005;49(3):895–902.

[49] Bisland SK, Chien C, Wilson BC, et al. Pre-clinical in vitro and in vivo studies to examine the potential use of photodynamic therapy in the treatment of osteomyelitis. Photochem Photobiol Sci 2006;5(1): 31–8.

[50] Kamp H, Tietz HJ, Lutz M, et al. Antifungal effect of 5-aminolevulinic acid PDT in *Trichophyton rubrum.* Mycoses 2005;48(2):101–7.

[51] de Souza SC, Junqueira JC, Balducci I, et al. Photosensitization of different *Candida* species by low power laser light. J Photochem Photobiol B 2006; 83(1):34–8.

[52] Teichert MC, Jones JW, Usacheva MN, et al. Treatment of oral candidiasis with methylene blue-mediated photodynamic therapy in an immunodeficient murine model. Oral Surg Oral Med Oral Pathol Oral Radiol Endod 2002;93(2):155–60.

[53] Calzavara-Pinton PG, Venturini M, Capezzera R, et al. Photodynamic therapy of interdigital mycoses of the feet with topical application of 5-aminolevulinic acid. Photodermatol Photoimmunol Photomed 2004;20(3):144–7.

[54] Gold MH, Boring MM, Bridges TM, et al. The successful use of ALA-PDT in the treatment of recalcitran molluscum contagiosum. J Drugs Dermatol 2004;3(2):187–90.

[55] Smetana Z, Ben-Hur E, Mendelson E, et al. Herpes simplex virus proteins are damaged following photodynamic inactivation with phthalocyanines. J Photochem Photobiol B 1998;44(1):77–83.

[56] Smetana Z, Malik Z, Orenstein A, et al. Treatment of viral infections with 5-aminolevulinic acid and light. Lasers Surg Med 1997;21(4):351–8.

[57] Jori G. Photodynamic therapy of microbial infections: state of the art and perspectives. J Environ Pathol Toxicol Oncol 2006;25(1–2):505–20.

[58] Grossman M, Anderson A. Presented at 1996 American Society for Laser Medicine and Surgery Annual Meeting.

[59] Parlette EC. Red light laser photodynamic therapy of Bowen's disease. J Drugs Dermatol 2004;3(6): S22–4.

ELSEVIER
SAUNDERS

Dermatol Clin 25 (2007) 111–118

DERMATOLOGIC
CLINICS

Incorporating Photodynamic Therapy into a Medical and Cosmetic Dermatology Practice

Dore J. Gilbert, MD[a,b,*]

[a]Newport Dermatology and Laser Associates, 1441 Avacado, Suite 806, Newport Beach, CA 92660, USA
[b]University of California, Irvine, Irvine, CA 92697, USA

Although shown to enhance both clinical and cosmetic outcomes of patients with many skin diseases [1,2], photodynamic therapy (PDT) has not been implemented by most dermatologists. One reason is that the most extensively studied photosensitizing agent, 5-aminolevulinic acid (ALA) (Levulan Kerastick, DUSA Pharmaceuticals, Wilmington, Massachusetts), has received Food and Drug Administration (FDA) clearance for only nonhypertrophic actinic keratoses (AK) of the face and scalp. Other reasons include limited reimbursement for AK by ALA-PDT, lack of insurance coverage for acne vulgaris and other conditions treatable by ALA-PDT, and concern about patient downtime and phototoxicity [3].

Clinical guidelines for the use of ALA-PDT have recently been published [3], but information on how to implement ALA-PDT is limited. This article describes how and why the author introduced ALA-PDT to his patients, what factors he considered in deciding whether to implement ALA-PDT, how he introduced ALA-PDT to new and existing patients, and the financial impact of the technique on the author's practice. The review also considers pretreatment and posttreatment care, treatment parameters, and risks associated with ALA-PDT. The author uses ALA-PDT for the treatment of AK, nonmelanoma skin cancer, acne vulgaris, sebaceous hyperplasia, and photodamage.

Principles of 5-aminolevulinic acid photodynamic therapy

To have a therapeutic or cosmetic effect, ALA-PDT requires a (1) topically administered photosensitizing agent that accumulates more readily in target tissue than in normal, healthy tissue; (2) a light source to activate photosensitizer; and (3) molecular oxygen. After entering tissue through the stratum corneum, ALA is converted to protoporphyrin IX (PpIX), which in the presence of light of wavelengths absorbed by PpIX (Fig. 1) is converted to singlet oxygen, a metastable intermediate believed to cause necrosis in the target tissue without damaging surrounding tissue [4,5]. This selectivity is largely responsible for the safety and efficacy of ALA-PDT [6,7].

In general, long wavelengths of light (up to 850 nm) [8] penetrate deeper into tissue than short wavelengths of light [9]. Intense pulsed light (IPL) and pulsed dye laser (PDL) systems emit wavelengths with the deepest penetration. With PDLs, practitioners can stack pulses to treat troublesome lesions more effectively. Because ALA diffusion and subsequent cellular destruction are limited to the epidermis [7] and sebaceous glands [10], healing occurs rapidly and the risks of scarring and infection are minimal [7,11].

Another major advantage of ALA-PDT is that many light or laser sources can be used to activate ALA-induced PpIX (Table 1) [2,3]. For this reason, physicians with one or more light sources may already have the necessary in-office equipment to implement ALA-PDT. Blue light (BLU-U, DUSA Pharmaceuticals, Wilmington, Massachusetts) provides light at 417 nm, the maximum absorption peak of ALA-induced PpIX. The BLU-U is the only FDA-cleared light source for use in

The author has received equipment from Dusa Pharmaceuticals for research purposes. He has also served as a funded speaker.

* Newport Dermatology and Laser Associates, 1441 Avocado, Suite 806, Newport Beach, CA 92660.

E-mail address: lazrdoc@pacbell.net.

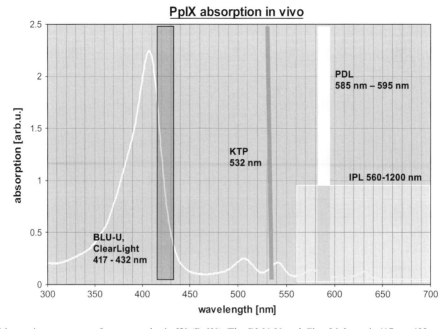

Fig. 1. Absorption spectrum of protoporphyrin IX (PpIX). The BLU-U and ClearLight emit 417- to 432-nm light, the wavelength range of maximum absorption by PpIX. Smaller PpIX absorption peaks appear at larger wavelengths that, although absorbed less by PpIX, are useful in photodynamic therapy because penetration of longer-wavelength light into the skin is deeper than at the 417- to 432-nm range. The potassium titanyl phosphate (KTP) laser emits 532-nm light, the pulsed dye laser (PDL) emits 585- to 595-nm light, and intense pulsed light (IPL) provides 560- to 1200-nm broadband light. Because each of these wavelengths (or wavelength ranges) is absorbed by PpIX, each of these devices can be used to activate PpIX in photodynamic therapy. (*From* Nestor MS, Gold MH, Kauvar AN, et al. The use of photodynamic therapy in dermatology: results of a consensus conference. J Drugs Dermatol 2006;5:140–54; with permission.)

ALA-PDT at the time of this writing. The author has found blue light to be very effective in a variety of applications.

Two photosensitizing agents are commercially available for PDT: ALA and methyl aminolevulinate (Metvix, PhotoCure ASA, Oslo, Norway). Methyl aminolevulinate is approved in Europe for the treatment of AK of the face and scalp and basal cell carcinoma unsuitable for conventional therapy. The FDA cleared Metvix for AK in 2004, but the product is not yet available in the United States. Because the author practices in the United States, this article focuses only on implementing PDT with ALA.

Reasons to implement 5-aminolevulinic acid photodynamic therapy

New therapeutic option

Actinic keratoses

ALA-PDT is an excellent primary and adjunctive therapy for AK. For example, 5-fluorouracil and other topical medications may require up to 16 weeks of therapy, during which treated areas are erythematous. With ALA-PDT, posttreatment erythema subsides within 1 week unless multiple treatments are necessary. In the latter case, treatment sessions may be spaced so that erythema does not compromise patient lifestyles. The author has shown that 5-fluorouracil may be used in sequential combination with single-session ALA-PDT with IPL for the treatment of AK [12]. With this combination, 90% of treated AKs had resolved in 14 of 15 patients at 1 month and 1 year posttreatment and erythema had resolved within 7 to 10 days. Given a choice, most patients choose a 1-week therapy that produces redness and scaling over the alternative (5-fluorouracil), in which redness lasts 4 weeks. ALA-PDT has also been successful in the treatment of AK over large surfaces [13–16].

Acne vulgaris and sebaceous skin

Many patients with acne vulgaris wish to avoid prolonged use of antibiotics. They also prefer an

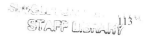

Table 1
Consensus recommendations for light sources, number of treatments, and treatment intervals for photodynamic therapy with 5-aminolevulinic acid

Dermatologic condition	Light source (preferred/ alternate/other)	No. of treatments (interval)	Comment
Actinic keratoses, superficial basal cell carcinoma	Blue/PDL[a], IPL[b]/green, yellow, red	1–2 (3–5 or 2 wk) [c]	
Photodamage or cosmetic enhancement	IPL[b] (blue for skin type VI)/Blue, PDL[a]/green, yellow[d]	At least 2 (2–4 or 1 wk) [c], depending on severity of damage	Typically five treatments at 2–3 wk intervals; three treatments include ALA
Acne vulgaris	PDL → blue (5 min)/blue (8 min)/green, red, IPL, yellow	1–3 (2–3 wk)[e]	Treat flares immediately; 6–12 mo clearance typical
Sebaceous skin, rosacea, rhinophyma	PDL[f], blue/IPL[b]/green[f], yellow, red	1–2 (3–5 or 2 wk) [c]	

"Preferred" sources produce the most significant response for the lesion type and may cause response without ALA (ie, IPL for photodamage, PDL for acne vulgaris).

"Alternate" sources result in substantial effectiveness against the lesion type.

"Other" sources have unproved effectiveness against the lesion type (ie, 532-nm light for acne vulgaris).

Abbreviations: ALA, aminolevulinic acid; IPL, intense pulsed light; PDL, pulsed dye laser.

[a] Fluences that avoid bruising.

[b] Standard photorejuvenation settings by patient type.

[c] Increase ALA incubation time if necessary in second and subsequent treatments.

[d] Optimum is IPL, PDL, or green (532 nm) followed by blue light for 5 min. (The author of this paper recommends 10 min of blue light treatment.)

[e] For skin types IV–VI, ALA incubated 30 min for first treatment.

[f] Double or triple pulsing on lesion recommended.

Adapted from Nestor MS, Gold MH, Kauvar AN, et al. The use of photodynamic therapy in dermatology: results of a consensus conference. J Drugs Dermatol 2006;5:140–54; with permission.

alternative to isotretinoin because of concern regarding isotretinoin's side effects and new regulations that limit its use. In addition, patients with erythematous scars (often from acne vulgaris) notice improvement and a return of their skin to a normal color after ALA-PDT. The use of ALA-PDT in the treatment of sebaceous disorders has been reviewed [3].

Emerging applications

ALA-PDT has been used to treat a variety of difficult-to-treat cutaneous disorders, including hidradenitis suppurativa, molluscum contagiosum, cutaneous T-cell lymphoma, cutaneous leishmaniasis, extramammary Paget's disease, Hailey-Hailey disease, keratoacanthoma, keratosis pilaris, mycosis fungoides, perioral dermatitis, nevus sebaceous, psoriasis, localized scleroderma, and warts [3].

Cosmetic benefits

ALA-PDT offers cosmetic benefits when used alone or in combination with other therapies [2].

Cosmetic improvement is equivalent to that obtained with a 30% trichlorocetic acid peel, but healing is more rapid and serious side effects (eg, scarring) occur less frequently [11]. In the author's experience, significant improvements in hyperpigmentation, erythema, photodamage, and fine lines and reductions in pore size are often visible after ALA-PDT.

Enhanced effects of intense pulsed light

When used in combination with IPL, PDT increases turnover of pigmented cells and promotes reduction of telangiectasias (decreasing erythema) in the author's experience. Fewer IPL treatments are required for photorejuvenation and overall cosmetic appearance improves.

Financial benefits

In the author's practice, fees for ALA-PDT range from $300 to $1000 per treatment session, depending on the light source and the amount of photosensitizing agent required for the procedure.

Adding ALA-PDT has significantly increased practice revenue, especially when the technique is used for cosmetic purposes. Patients who experience ALA-PDT's cosmetic benefits often inquire about botulinum toxin injections, dermal filler injections, leg-vein removal, Photofacial, and cosmetic surgical procedures.

The learning curve

ALA-PDT is easy to perform and requires no additional staff members. Training is simple, especially when the light source for activation is in the physician's office and being used for other procedures. If a light source must be purchased, the physician can begin training staff as soon as the physician becomes comfortable in its use.

Physicians new to ALA-PDT should be as consistent as possible with ALA incubation times (30–60 minutes) and light activation technique. AK is the easiest condition to treat, whereas acne vulgaris is the most difficult because of the young age of most patients, school absences, and the number of treatment sessions required.

Costs and reimbursement

Light sources needed to activate ALA-induced PpIX are priced from $8000 for blue light to $100,000 for IPL systems. Continuous and pulsed light-emitting diodes for red and blue wavelengths cost approximately $30,000. High-quality digital imaging equipment for photographic documentation of patient responses costs $4000 to $6000 or more.

The major consumable in ALA-PDT is the photosensitizing agent, ALA. A Levulan Kerastick costs approximately $94 and a single treatment session requires one or two Kerasticks. Other consumables vary with the light source and their costs are negligible, especially when the light source is blue light.

The composition and terminology of the Levulan Kerastick are quoted below from the package insert:

> Levulan Kerastick (aminolevulinic acid HCl) for Topical Solution, 20%, contains the hydrochloride salt of ALA. The Levulan Kerastick for Topical Solution applicator is a two component system consisting of a plastic tube containing two sealed glass ampules and an applicator tip. One ampule contains 1.5 mL of solution vehicle comprising alcohol USP (ethanol content = 48% v/v), water, laureth-4, isopropyl alcohol,

and polyethylene glycol. The other ampule contains 354 mg of ALA HCl as a dry solid. The applicator tube is enclosed in a protective cardboard sleeve and cap. The 20% topical solution is prepared just before the time of use by breaking the ampules and mixing the contents by shaking the Levulan Kerastick applicator. The term "ALA HCl" refers to unformulated active ingredient, "Levulan Kerastick for Topical Solution" refers to the drug product in its unmixed state, "Levulan Kerastick Topical Solution" refers to the mixed drug product (in the applicator tube or after application), and "Levulan Kerastick" refers to the applicator only.

Insurance companies cover only FDA-cleared indications for ALA-PDT, such as AK. The use of Levulan or BLU-U for the treatment of conditions other than AK (acne vulgaris, photodamage, sebaceous hyperplasia, and rosacea) is considered off-label and usually not covered. Coverage for off-label indications, however, may be possible through direct involvement of the physician. For best results, the physician should contact the patient's insurance carrier directly and inquire about precertification for treatment of a specific patient. The likelihood of reimbursement differs among regions of the United States and among insurance companies.

Physical requirements

No office space is necessary other than the space required for a light source. The BLU-U requires approximately 2 sq ft and fits into the corner of a room. Light-emitting diode units can be placed on a desk. Most light sources require 110 V, so special wiring is not necessary.

Patients and scheduling

Patients suitable for ALA-PDT are willing to tolerate the down time and have enough disposable income for cosmetic treatments. Typical candidates have diffuse AK and photodamaged skin with red or brown discoloration. Patients who have failed oral and topical medications for acne vulgaris are also excellent candidates for ALA-PDT.

PDT sessions should be scheduled late in the afternoon to reduce the likelihood of posttreatment exposure to the sun's ultraviolet radiation. Treatments given on Thursday or Friday permit patients to recover from posttreatment erythema and scaling during the weekend so they can return to work the following Monday. Men can often resume shaving and women can apply makeup by the fifth day after treatment.

Introducing photodynamic therapy to patients

In the author's practice, the physician, a registered nurse, or both describe the efficacy and safety of ALA-PDT to patients. Registered nurses, for example, explain ALA-PDT to patients undergoing Photofacial treatments, whereas the physician discusses ALA-PDT as a treatment option to patients with AK or acne vulgaris. Educational materials should include photos of patients treated before and after ALA-PDT.

As with any procedure, patients must be counseled about possible adverse effects in advance, even though the potential side effects with ALA-PDT are mild and temporary. They must also be shown photos of mild and severe reactions to the procedure. Postprocedural instructions should be detailed and specific and patients should be encouraged to contact the physician's office with questions.

Preparing patients for treatment

The author's pretreatment protocol is outlined in Box 1.

This protocol is in agreement with ALA-PDT consensus guidelines [3].

Treatment procedure

In patients who have never received ALA-PDT, ALA should remain in contact with the target area for approximately 1 hour for most skin conditions. Longer incubation periods may be required in patients who have not responded to earlier treatment as shown by the absence of significant erythema or less-than-anticipated cosmetic improvement, or in patients who seek treatment of severe AK, superficial basal cell carcinoma, or squamous cell carcinoma. In these two patient groups, 2 to 3 hours or overnight ALA incubation may be necessary to achieve the desired results.

For a given patient, responses in previous treatment sessions may be used as a guide for adjusting treatment parameters in subsequent sessions. For example, if a patient had minimal erythema after the most recent session, the physician may increase the fluence or ALA incubation time in the next treatment session.

Box 1. ALA-PDT pretreatment protocol

1. Photograph the patient with both digital and Polaroid cameras. Place photographs on the patient's chart.
2. Instruct patient to continue topical or systemic medications.
3. Treat the target area with a short course of imiquimod or 5-fluorouracil if desired.
4. Wash the target area with soap and water or alcohol.
5. Perform either single-pass microdermabrasion, acetone scrub, or both to remove the keratin layer and increase ALA penetration. In teenaged patients, scrub to the patient's comfort level.
6. Gently crush ALA ampules with the fingers and shake the Kerastick for approximately 3 minutes, keeping the sponge end up.
7. Apply ALA liberally to the skin, using extra pressure to the target lesions. Spread the solution uniformly with gloved fingertips. Avoid mucous membranes.
8. Allow ALA to incubate for at least 30 to 60 minutes.
9. Remove ALA with soap and water only if using large amounts of gel during IPL treatment. Otherwise, leave ALA on the skin.
10. Wash the patient's face after treatment is completed.

In the author's practice, treatment parameters for AK by ALA-PDT include 1-hour ALA incubation; IPL (Lumenis One, Lumenis) activation with a 560-nm filter using 16 J/cm^2 fluence; double 4-millisecond pulsing; and 20-millisecond delay at the time of this writing. The author usually treats IPL-exposed areas with blue light for an additional 10 minutes unless patient discomfort becomes excessive. Patients receiving blue light treatment are given a hand fan to reduce discomfort. Alternatively, IPL pulse durations may be lengthened to increase contact time with skin.

Light-emitting diode systems have also been very effective in ALA-PDT (Table 2). Time of

Table 2
Duration of irradiation with light emitting diode systems in aminolevulinic acid photodynamic therapy for acne vulgaris, photodamage, actinic keratoses, and other applications

LED device	Duration (min)
Omnilux Red[a]	15
Omnilux Blue[a]	12
GentleWaves[b] (red)	14
GentleWaves[b] (yellow)	15

   [a] Alderm LLC, Irvine, California.
   [b] Light BioScience LLC, Virginia Beach, Virginia.

exposure to light-emitting diode energy varies from 12 to 15 minutes.

The author recently used ALA-PDT for the treatment of severe pustular and cystic acne vulgaris. ALA incubation time was 30 to 60 minutes and ALA-induced PpIX was activated by PDL (V-star, Cynosure) and blue light systems. Our V-star settings included 12-mm spot size, 10-millisecond pulse duration, and 3 to 5 J/cm^2. A major advantage of PDL treatment is that pulses can be stacked onto difficult target areas.

Evaluating results

In the author's practice, responses of AK patients to ALA-PDT are evaluated 1 week, 1 month, and even 1 year after treatment. Improvement is usually noticeable at 1 month. Patients with acne vulgaris are treated once monthly for 4 months, then treated again as needed. Visible

improvement usually requires 2 to 4 monthly treatments. Patients with sebaceous hyperplasia receive a single treatment with 1-month follow-up.

Adverse effects

The author has experienced minimal adverse effects with ALA-PDT and all are temporary. Patient education and compliance are vital to avoid phototoxic reactions for 2 weeks after ALA-PDT. Anesthesia during treatment is not necessary for most patients.

The risks of bacterial infection, exacerbation of herpetic infections, persistent erythema, postinflammatory hyperpigmentation or hypopigmentation, and hypertrophic scars (the author has never seen one attributable to ALA-PDT), however, should be considered. Bacterial infection is managed with appropriate antibiotics and cleansing. Patients with a history of herpetic infection should be treated with prophylactic antiviral medications (valacyclovir, 1 g twice a day, 1 day before, the day of, and the day after ALA-PDT). Erythema may be treated with topical steroids and hyperpigmentation with hydroquinones. Rare hypertrophic scars are treated with intralesional steroids and PDL therapy. Adverse effects and their treatments are summarized in Table 3.

Posttreatment care

Compared with carbon-dioxide and Er:YAG laser therapy, ALA-PDT recovery time is short. Because ALA-PDT causes minimal damage to the dermis, epidermal re-epithelization occurs quickly

Table 3
Adverse effects of photodynamic therapy with 5-aminolevulinic acid

Adverse effect	Frequency (%)	Duration (d)	Treatment
Erythema	85	3–7	Hydrocortisone ointment
Flakiness	85	3–4	Moisturizer
Edema	75	1–4	Ice pack
Crusting	50	2–3	Water and vinegar soaks
Oozing or vesiculation	25	2–3	Vinegar soaks
Pain	20	1–2	Over-the counter analgesic
Hyperpigmentation	5	14	—
Blistering	1	2–5	Ice pack

   From Gilbert DJ. Post-treatment care for photodynamic therapy with topical 5-aminolevulinic acid. US dermatology 2006. London: Touch Briefings; 2006. p. 85–7; with permission.

[7]. The author's protocol for post–ALA-PDT care for all light sources and types of lesions is shown in Box 2.

Redness, scaling, and slight swelling are common during the first 12 hours after treatment. During the next 24 hours, swelling (most pronounced around the eyes) continues and redness may increase. Ice packs reduce discomfort and swelling. Skin reactivity increases with long ALA incubation time [11].

Patients should avoid exposure to the sun for the first 24 to 48 hours after ALA-PDT [3]. During this period, residual ALA is converted to PpIX and residual PpIX clears from skin. If residual PpIX is exposed to UV radiation, it becomes activated and the patient experiences itching, burning, and other manifestations of phototoxicity [7]. The application of titanium dioxide–zinc oxide has been recommended to block UVA and UVB light [3].

During days 2 through 7, patients should continue with ice packs and pain medication and should treat blistered, edematous areas (see Box 2). Blisters have been reported in patients receiving ALA-PDT with red light [17]. Because new epidermal cells are sensitive to sunlight, patients should protect the treated areas from sun for 2 weeks after treatment. When redness and scaling are no longer present (4–5 days after treatment), healing is complete. Most patients comply with these instructions [11].

In the author's experience, ALA-PDT wound severity increases with ALA incubation time, fluence, and number of passes. Wound severity also depends on the light source and activation wavelength [11].

Box 2. Posttreatment home care after PDT

Day of ALA-PDT
- Apply ice packs to treated areas
- Take pain medication as needed
- Avoid sun exposure for 24 hours
  - Stay indoors
  - Apply sunscreen (to all exposed skin, not just treated area)
  - Wear a hat
- Apply hydrocortisone (1%) ointment to treated area
- Take a shower if desired

Days 2 to 7
- Continue pain medication and ice packs as needed
- Protect treated area from sun exposure
- If blisters develop
  1. Soak in white vinegar solution (1 teaspoon vinegar in 1 cup cold water)
  2. Apply ice over vinegar-soaked areas for 20 minutes
  3. Pat areas dry
  4. Apply petrolatum or hydrocortisone (1%) ointment
  5. Repeat steps 1 to 4 at 4- to 6-hour intervals during waking hours
  6. Apply petrolatum (Aquaphor) or hydrocortisone (1%) ointment twice daily as needed

Day 7
- Apply makeup if healing is complete, use moisturizer before applying makeup
- Protect treated area from sun exposure (for 2 weeks total after treatment)
- Apply sun block (at least 30 SPF) to treated area during sun exposure for 2 weeks after treatment
- If treated area is red after crusting has subsided, apply green-based cover-up to hide redness

---

Adapted from Gilbert DJ. Post-treatment care for photodynamic therapy with topical 5-aminolevulinic acid. In: US dermatology 2006. London: Touch Briefings; 2006. p. 85–7.

Summary

ALA-PDT is a safe, effective, and easy-to-perform procedure for the treatment of a variety of cutaneous conditions. Pretreatment and post-treatment procedures are straightforward and well documented. Adverse effects are mild, temporary, and easily managed. Light sources may already be available in physicians' offices or may be purchased for $8000. Cosmetic benefits of ALA-PDT encourage patients to seek additional cosmetic treatments, increasing practice revenue.

References

[1] Taub AF. Photodynamic therapy in dermatology: history and horizons. J Drugs Dermatol 2004;3:8S–25S.

[2] Gold MH, Goldman MP. 5-aminolevulinic acid photodynamic therapy: where we have been and where we are going. Dermatol Surg 2004;30:1077–83.

[3] Nestor MS, Gold MH, Kauvar AN, et al. The use of photodynamic therapy in dermatology: results of a consensus conference. J Drugs Dermatol 2006;5:140–54.

[4] Weishaupt KR, Gomer CJ, Dougherty TJ. Identification of singlet oxygen as the cytotoxic agent in photoinactivation of a murine tumor. Cancer Res 1976;36(7 pt 1):2326–9.

[5] Niedre MJ, Yu CS, Patterson MS, et al. Singlet oxygen luminescence as an in vivo photodynamic therapy dose metric: validation in normal mouse skin with topical amino-levulinic acid. Br J Cancer 2005;92:298–304.

[6] Kennedy JC, Pottier RH, Pross DC. Photodynamic therapy with endogenous protoporphyrin IX: basic principles and present clinical experience. J Photochem Photobiol B 1990;6:143–8.

[7] Kennedy J, Pottier R. Endogenous protoporphyrin IX, a clinically useful photosensitizer for photodynamic therapy. J Photochem Photobiol B 1992;14:275–92.

[8] Kalka K, Merk H, Mukhtar H. Photodynamic therapy in dermatology. J Am Acad Dermatol 2000;42:389–413.

[9] Wilson BC, Patterson MS. The physics of photodynamic therapy. Phys Med Biol 1986;31:327–60.

[10] Hongcharu W, Taylor C, Chang Y, et al. Topical ALA-photodynamic therapy for the treatment of acne vulgaris. J Invest Dermatol 2000;115:183–92.

[11] Gilbert DJ. Post-treatment care for photodynamic therapy with topical 5-aminolevulinic acid. In: US dermatology 2006. London: Touch Briefings; 2006. p. 85–7.

[12] Gilbert DJ. Treatment of actinic keratoses with sequential combination of 5-fluorouracil and photodynamic therapy. J Drugs Dermatol 2005;4:161–3.

[13] Smith S, Piacquadio D, Morhenn V, et al. Short incubation PDT versus 5-FU in treating actinic keratoses. J Drugs Dermatol 2003;2:629–35.

[14] Bissonette R, Bergeron A, Liu Y. Large surface photodynamic therapy with aminolevulinic acid: treatment of actinic keratoses and beyond. J Drugs Dermatol 2004;3(1 Suppl):26S–31S.

[15] Liu Y, Viau G, Bissonette R. Multiple large-surface photodynamic therapy sessions with topical or systemic aminolevulinic acid and blue light in UV-exposed hairless mice. J Cutan Med Surg 2004;8:131–9.

[16] Touma D, Yaar M, Whitehead S, et al. A trial of short incubation, broad-area photodynamic therapy for facial actinic keratoses and diffuse photodamage. Arch Dermatol 2004;140:33–40.

[17] Fijan S, Honigsmann H, Ortel B. Photodynamic therapy of epithelial skin tumours using delta-aminolaevulinic acid and desferrioxamine. Br J Dermatol 1995;133:282–8.

Photodynamic Therapy in Dermatology: the Next Five Years

Michael H. Gold, MD[a,b,*]

[a]*Gold Skin Care Center, Tennessee Clinical Research Center, 2000 Richard Jones Road,
Suite 220, Nashville, TN 37215, USA*
[b]*Vanderbilt University Medical School, Vanderbilt University Nursing School,
Nashville, TN 37215, USA*

The next 5 years for the study of photodynamic therapy (PDT) seem to be very bright. This issue introduces the reader to where the field has been with PDT in the past, where PDT is at the present time, and has given some insights as to where PDT will be in the future.

The following are solely my perceptions and ideas as to where PDT is heading in dermatology. The comments are mine and mine alone. Others have different opinions and that is okay, because continued dialog and continued study in this field only enhance the use of PDT.

Currently in the United States there is only one photosensitizer available, 20% 5-aminolevulinic acid (ALA). It has Food and Drug Administration clearance for the treatment of nonhyperkeratotic actinic keratoses (AKs) of the face and scalp using a blue light source after a drug incubation of 14 to 18 hours. Clinical studies, presented in this issue, have shown its effectiveness in treating AKs. Further clinical investigations by forward-thinking clinicians and researchers have demonstrated that by using a shorter contact mode for ALA, efficacy can be maintained and improvements clinically can be obtained. Improvements in AKs and photorejuvenation parameters are seen with short-contact, full-face ALA applications and the use of a variety of blue light sources, and other lasers and light sources, which deliver light energy in the absorption spectrum of the active form of ALA in the skin, protoporphyrin IX. These lasers and light sources include the KTP lasers, the long-pulsed pulsed dye lasers, and the intense-pulsed light sources. Improvement in patients with moderate to severe inflammatory acne vulgaris, sebaceous gland hyperplasia, and hidradenitis suppurativa also has been shown with short-contact ALA-PDT therapy. The use of ALA-PDT in all but what has originally been approved by the FDA is considered off-label use of ALA-PDT, but has become the standard of care in many clinical settings around the United States.

In Europe, the methyl ester of ALA is currently the drug of choice for use in PDT. Its predominant indication is for the treatment of nonhyperkeratotic AKs of the face and scalp and superficial nonmelanoma skin cancers unsuitable for conventional therapy. Its use is recommended with 3-hour drug incubation under occlusion and best used with a red light source at 630 nm. Several clinical investigators have begun to look at the use of this methyl ester in the treatment of photorejuvenation, inflammatory acne vulgaris, and in hidradenitis suppurativa. At the time of this writing, the methyl ester of ALA is FDA approved for the treatment of AKs in the United States, but is currently not yet marketed or available in this country.

Eventually, both of the ALA products and perhaps other esters as well will find their niches

Dr. Gold is a consultant for Dusa Pharmaceuticals, speaks on their behalf, receives honoraria, and performs research on their behalf. Dr. Gold is also a consultant for numerous pharmaceutical and device companies and performs research on their behalf.

* Gold Skin Care Center, Tennessee Clinical Research Center, 2000 Richard Jones Road, Suite 220, Nashville, TN 37215.

   E-mail address: goldskin@goldskincare.com.

for a variety of skin disorders dermatologists treat on a regular basis. PDT will become "global." If the specialty of PDT is to continue to grow, clinicians have to determine which ALA product works best for which condition and learn how to maximize the therapy with each of the products available. For instance, in the United States, clinicians have studied and published that short-contact, full-face therapy works just as well as the original descriptions of long drug incubation. Not only can one use blue light, but also a variety of lasers and light sources that many already have in the office settings to make the therapy available to more and more clinicians. Most of these studies have shown that the treatments are tolerated well, with very little, if any, downtime associated with the therapy.

In Europe, research is just beginning on photorejuvenation, acne vulgaris, and other indications. Preliminary data, although encouraging from an end point efficacy standpoint, have been associated with a great deal of adverse effects as a result of the therapy, including what has been called the "PDT effect," or downtime with healing, something that most patients do not want when coming to a physician for this type of therapy. Further research with shorter-contact methyl ALA therapy has to be performed, in manners similar to United States studies, to determine if methyl ALA works as well for these "cosmetic" indications.

Research on both of the products will determine which product works best for each specific indication. Perhaps the research will show that with short-contact, full-face therapy works similarly with both of the currently available products. Then other factors, such as cost of the drugs and pharmaceutical support of the specialties, will play a role in which drug is used when. Currently, I believe that they will play out as follows:

AKs: ALA and methyl ALA equal
AKs and photorejuvenation: ALA > methyl ALA
Bowen's disease: methyl ALA
Nonmelanoma skin cancers: methyl ALA
Acne vulgaris: ALA > methyl ALA
Sebaceous gland hyperplasia: ALA
Hidradenitis suppurativa: ALA > methyl ALA
Chemoprevention: ALA and methyl ALA equal

The last item on this list is to me the most important. Chemoprevention represents the most important clinical concern that PDT can definitely affect and where a great deal of future research endeavors need to be centered. Although not as "sexy" as some of the other indications, chemoprevention with these agents offers a topical therapy for patients that will affect their lives for as long as they live. As an antidote, and on a personal note, I have been following my own father for many years with diffuse actinic damage and numerous AKs and a history of numerous skin cancers. He has had many ALA-PDT treatments and has had the number of skin cancers found and treated reduced to one in the past 7 years, something that I truly relate to having treated him with ALA-PDT until clear in the late 1990s and then doing maintenance therapy on a two to three times per year basis since that time. He is a walking example of the chemoprevention potential of PDT. It is very fortunate that in the field of PDT there are wonderful researchers studying the affects of PDT in animal models, in patients with multiple skin cancers, and in immunosuppressed individuals to determine fully the chemoprevention potentials of both ALA and the methyl ester of ALA. I again encourage pharmaceutical companies to continue funding for these incredibly worthwhile research endeavors and for clinicians to ensure that these researchers have open forums to present their data, which I believe are more important than any other potential use of ALA-PDT.

Finally, clinicians must continue to strive to make PDT a global subspecialty of dermatology. It should not be European PDT and the United States PDT, but global PDT looking for the best uses of the products to help patients. Clinicians need to combine resources and strengths, and begin to do collaborative clinical trials to optimize PDT for all. If this can be accomplished, then there will truly be global PDT and a force that provides new and exciting therapies for patients who ultimately benefit from clinicians' knowledge and ingenuity.

Good luck to all who use PDT and continued success to those who study PDT.

ELSEVIER
SAUNDERS

Dermatol Clin 25 (2007) 121–125

DERMATOLOGIC
CLINICS

Index

Note: Page numbers of article titles are in **boldface** type.

Moving?

Make sure your subscription moves with you!

To notify us of your new address, find your **Clinics Account Number** (located on your mailing label above your name), and contact customer service at:

E-mail: elspcs@elsevier.com

800-654-2452 (subscribers in the U.S. & Canada)
407-345-4000 (subscribers outside of the U.S. & Canada)

Fax number: 407-363-9661

Elsevier Periodicals Customer Service
6277 Sea Harbor Drive
Orlando, FL 32887-4800

*To ensure uninterrupted delivery of your subscription, please notify us at least 4 weeks in advance of move.

ELSEVIER